The **DASH Diet**

# 30-MINUTE
# COOKBOOK

Quick and Easy Recipes
to Help You Lose Your Salt
Habit and Lose Weight

## CHRISTY ELLINGSWORTH

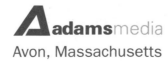

Avon, Massachusetts

Published by

Adams Media, a division of F+W Media, Inc.

57 Littlefield Street, Avon, MA 02322. U.S.A.

www.adamsmedia.com

Contains material adapted from *The Everything® DASH Diet Cookbook* by Christy Ellingsworth and Murdoc Khaleghi, MD, copyright © 2012 by F+W Media, Inc., ISBN 10: 1-4405-4353-4, ISBN 13: 978-1-4405-4353-1.

ISBN 10: 1-4405-9072-9

ISBN 13: 978-1-4405-9072-6

eISBN 10: 1-4405-9073-7

eISBN 13: 978-1-4405-9073-3

Printed in the United States of America.

10   9   8   7   6   5   4   3   2   1

The information in this book should not be used for diagnosing or treating any health problem. Not all diet and exercise plans suit everyone. You should always consult a trained medical professional before starting a diet, taking any form of medication, or embarking on any fitness or weight-training program. The author and publisher disclaim any liability arising directly or indirectly from the use of this book.

Always follow safety and commonsense cooking protocol while using kitchen utensils, operating ovens and stoves, and handling uncooked food. If children are assisting in the preparation of any recipe, they should always be supervised by an adult.

Cover design by Sylvia McArdle.

Cover images © Michael Gray/123RF; Larysa Kryvoshapka/123RF; serezniy/123RF; iStockphoto.com/pumatokoh; AbbieImages.

*This book is available at quantity discounts for bulk purchases.*

*For information, please call 1-800-289-0963.*

## Chapter 5: Snacks and Drinks . . . . . . . . . . . . . . . . . . 91

## Chapter 6: Appetizers and Side Dishes . . . . . . . . . . . . . 113

# Introduction

Are you looking for a natural way to improve your blood pressure, lower your cholesterol, and shed those extra pounds? With *The DASH Diet 30-Minute Cookbook*, you can achieve all your health goals with 175 scrumptious recipes that won't leave you feeling deprived—of taste *or* time.

The #1 diet in the United States, the DASH (Dietary Approaches to Stop Hypertension) diet is a balanced eating plan that is low in sodium and rich in fruits, vegetables, whole grains, and low-fat dairy products. It has been shown to reduce cholesterol, promote heart health, and lower blood pressure—all without the use of medications—in just fourteen days. As with many sensible eating plans, it has the added bonus of boosting weight loss and may also aid in the prevention of cancer, osteoporosis, and diabetes. In short, the DASH diet can help you live a longer, healthier life.

Developed around fresh, nourishing ingredients, the DASH diet lets you enjoy many of the same foods that you've always eaten. Yes, that even means eating mouthwatering desserts like Chocolate Cupcakes with Vanilla Frosting and Peanut Butter Chocolate Chip Blondies! From hearty breakfasts like Brown Sugar Cinnamon Oatmeal to savory snacks like Garlic Lovers Hummus each page provides you with step-by-step instructions for crafting dishes so flavorful you'll forget that they're part of a diet plan. Every recipe also includes nutritional stats to help keep you on track and encourage you to create meal plans that work for you and your taste buds.

These delicious dishes have also been designed with your busy lifestyle in mind and can be made—from start to finish—in thirty minutes or less. So you have dozens of meals, snacks, and treats that are ready to go when you are! No more slaving away in the kitchen trying to prepare a nutritious meal after a long day at work or stopping at the drive-thru because you don't have time to cook. With these tasty recipes, you'll have no excuse for not making yourself and your health a priority.

Like any diet, the DASH diet may be challenging at times, but don't give up! Remember that you have all the tools and recipes you need to quickly whip up a wholesome, mouthwatering meal whenever hunger hits. Success is just around the corner, so start building a healthier and happier lifestyle now with *The DASH Diet 30-Minute Cookbook*!

# CHAPTER 1

# The DASH Diet and How It Can Work for You

Unlike many fad diets, the DASH diet isn't a temporary fix, but a long-term solution for best health. It's an eating plan designed to heal your body by providing the nutrition you need without excess fat, sodium, and cholesterol. The DASH diet has the power to change your life dramatically, one delicious meal at a time.

## What Is the DASH Diet?

DASH is an acronym for Dietary Approaches to Stop Hypertension. The DASH diet is rich in fruits, vegetables, whole grains, and low-fat dairy products. Its emphasis isn't on deprivation, but on adaptation. The DASH diet aims to change the way people look at food, to educate them about their bodies, and to teach them to make healthy, sustainable choices.

The DASH diet was created to change lives by changing lifestyles. Unlike more restrictive diets, the DASH diet was designed to be approachable, and to be readily incorporated into people's lives. For the most part, you do not need to shop at special grocery stores or go through agonizing transition periods; you just need to start adjusting your food patterns, one step at a time.

The basics of the DASH diet are simple: Eat more fruits, vegetables, whole grains, and lean protein, and eat less saturated fat, salt, and sweets. It's a common-sense approach to health that really works.

## Show Me the Science

While other dietary plans may have little scientific support, the DASH diet has been proven through rigorous research. The National Institutes of Health, the premier governmental medical research agency of the United States, conducted two landmark trials showing that adherence to the DASH diet does indeed lower cholesterol and blood pressure. Other prestigious institutions, universities, and medical centers continue to study the positive effects of the DASH diet, offering new and exciting empirical evidence of its benefits.

The DASH diet was created to reduce hypertension in patients through diet, not drugs. Since its inception, it has been found to have many other health benefits, from decreasing the risk of cancer to reducing the risk of heart attack and stroke. It's no wonder that the DASH diet is the eating plan most often prescribed by physicians. And the news media, including *U.S. News & World Report*, repeatedly rank the DASH diet as the best diet overall.

## Hypertension

*Hypertension*, or high blood pressure, is often called a "silent killer" because its effects are often not felt until it's too late. Left unchecked, hypertension can, and often does, lead to a heart attack or stroke. These occur when plaque—a substance formed in the body—builds up in arteries, obstructing blood vessels and stifling the flow of blood and oxygen to the heart or brain. During a heart attack, the heart is unable to pump blood to the rest of the body; during a stroke, brain function is impaired and bodily control is lost, sometimes permanently. Heart attack and stroke are two of the leading causes of death in our society. But they are preventable. By limiting the formation of plaque in your arteries, you can reduce your risk of death and disability. To reduce plaque, you need to understand its cause and how your diet contributes to its formation.

**How Is Blood Pressure Measured?**
Blood pressure is measured in millimeters of mercury, or mmHg, and is given in the form of one number over another, for example: 100/70 mmHg. The first number, *systolic* blood pressure, represents the pressure exerted by your heart and blood when it is actively pumping. The second measurement, or *diastolic* blood pressure, represents the pressure between heartbeats when your heart is at rest. Blood pressure measurements are displayed by showing the systolic blood pressure *over* the diastolic blood pressure. People whose blood pressure measures between 90/60 mmHg and 140/90 mmHg have normal blood pressure; those above 140/90 mmHg have *hypertension* or high blood pressure.

*Blood pressure* indicates the amount of pressure required by your heart to circulate blood throughout your body. The higher your blood pressure, the harder your heart must work to do its job properly (i.e., deliver oxygen-rich blood to your cells). As blood pressure rises, so does the pressure within the blood vessels. This increase in pressure causes damage and, in combination with poor diet, leads to the formation of a sticky substance called plaque. Like plaster on walls, plaque accumulates and hardens along the lining of blood vessels, causing them to narrow. These narrowed vessels in turn make it harder for the heart to do its job. Blood pressure rises further. More damage is done. And if the diet remains poor, more plaque forms, eventually clogging arteries and causing heart attack or stroke. It's a vicious cycle, but it's preventable! By changing your diet, you can change—even save—your life. And it's never too late to start.

## Does the DASH Diet Really Work?

Studies of the DASH diet have consistently shown success in reducing blood pressure across test subjects. In general, people with normal blood pressure on the DASH diet have a reduction of about 6 mmHg in their systolic blood pressure and 3 mmHg in their diastolic blood pressure. And those with hypertension experience approximately *twice* this reduction in both systolic and diastolic blood pressures.

**Is the DASH Diet Just Another Fad?**
The DASH diet isn't a fad; it's nearly twenty years old and going strong! It was created in 1996 through the collaboration of researchers at several medical centers across the United States, including those of Duke and Johns Hopkins universities. The DASH diet is considered a respected, successful approach to combatting hypertension, reducing cholesterol, and maintaining heart health; all without medication.

The DASH diet can significantly reduce cardiovascular risk, with results comparable to many blood pressure medications. But unlike costly prescriptions with deleterious side effects, the only side effects of the DASH diet are improvements in blood pressure, cholesterol, cancer risk, and weight—all positives!

## Why Does It Work?

The DASH diet works because it's a *sustainable lifestyle*, not a traditional diet. The word "diet" conjures thoughts of temporary deprivation, but the DASH diet is the opposite. It's about teaching people how to eat properly, on a daily basis, so that they build healthy bodies. Rather than impose strict controls on food *content*, such as the number of grams of fat, the DASH diet is driven by guidelines to make smart food choices. When individuals understand the implications of their daily dietary decision making, they're much more likely to choose wisely. The lack of severe restriction allows individuals to transition gradually to a DASH diet, and to maintain that lifestyle once fully transitioned.

The ultimate goal of the DASH diet is to reduce the intake of harmful foods and to choose healthy substitutes instead. When you understand the damage that bad food does to your body, it makes you far less interested in eating it. And once you wean yourself from excess fat, cholesterol, sodium, and sugar, you will be amazed by how much better you feel! Bad food takes its toll in so many ways, not just silently with hypertension and heart disease, but also outwardly in your appearance, energy level, and enthusiasm for life. If you are feeling sluggish, consider what you last ate. Was it good for you? Or bad? Unless you are fueling your body with good food, it will fail you. The DASH diet isn't a strict dietary regimen, but rather a new way of seeing, appreciating, and consuming food.

## You Are What You Eat

To understand how the DASH diet affects your body, we must first discuss digestive physiology; that is, how the body breaks down food. The body absorbs three substances in food: protein, carbohydrates, and fat. Protein is used for building muscle mass and other tissue, while carbohydrates and fat are burned or stored for energy. The body first burns carbohydrates for fuel, and when those run low, it begins to break down fat.

## Calories and Fat

Carbohydrates, protein, and fat all possess a certain amount of energy, measured in calories. Carbohydrates and protein each contain 4 calories per gram, while fats have more than double that at 9 calories per gram. When you consume excess fat, therefore, you may *more than double* your caloric intake. And unless you expend those extra calories through work or exercise, they are stored in the body as fat. The greater the amount of stored fat, the harder its effects are on your body. The only way to break this cycle is to eat less fat, increase activity, or both.

## Carbohydrates

Despite a recent spate of bad press, carbohydrates remain the body's primary fuel source and are part of a healthy, balanced diet. Much of the criticism of carbohydrates lies in the fact that there are two distinct types, *complex* and *simple*, and they are not created equal. *Complex carbohydrates* are what you should be eating: things like fruits, vegetables, beans, low-fat dairy products, and whole-grain breads and pastas. During digestion, these complex carbohydrates are broken down more slowly than their inferior *simple* siblings. *Simple carbohydrates*, things like sweets and refined white flour products, are what you should avoid. Simple carbs are broken down quickly and absorbed into the bloodstream, giving you a sudden "sugar rush" that soon dissipates. When these types of carbohydrates are consumed in excess, they cause an increase in the release of *insulin*, a hormone that stores the carbohydrates as fat. Insulin spikes make you feel tired and promote *insulin resistance*, a precursor for diabetes. Avoiding simple carbohydrates and maintaining a steady, moderate consumption of complex carbohydrates will improve your energy and overall health.

## Sodium versus Salt

*Sodium* is a naturally occurring substance in food and helps regulate neurological and muscular function, as well as meet basic cellular needs. Some foods, such as fruit, contain very little natural sodium, while others, like shellfish, contain quite a lot. Humans require roughly 500 mg of sodium daily to maintain normal body processes. This daily requirement is easily met by eating a varied, healthy diet, and without the need of added salt.

*Salt* is not sodium. Salt is a naturally occurring compound that is harvested and used to enhance the taste of food. It contains sodium, yes, but it also contains chloride. Once added to food, salt cannot be taken away. Contrary to popular belief, you do not need salt to survive. It's a luxury, not a necessity.

When you eat salt, sodium is absorbed into your bloodstream, increasing the concentration of sodium in your blood relative to surrounding tissues. In an effort to maintain equilibrium across cells, fluid from the surrounding tissue passes via *osmosis* through cell membranes and into the bloodstream. This added fluid exerts greater pressure on your heart and blood vessels, effectively raising your blood pressure. In short, the more salt you eat, the higher your blood pressure will be. For those with hypertension, this is a particularly pressing issue (no pun intended).

## Cholesterol: The Good (HDL) and the Bad (LDL)

As mentioned previously, high blood pressure damages your blood vessels and leads to the formation of plaque, which can cause heart disease and stroke. Diet also plays a part in the formation of plaque, particularly with foods that are high in fat and cholesterol. *Cholesterol* is a waxy type of fat present in animal products. When you consume cholesterol it is absorbed into the bloodstream where it does one of two things. *Low-Density Lipoprotein (LDL)* or "bad" cholesterol, sticks to the walls of your arteries, contributing directly to the formation of plaque. *High-Density Lipoprotein (HDL)* or "good" cholesterol, acts as a sort of taxi, ferrying the bad LDL cholesterol out of the arteries.

**Not All Fat Is Bad!**
Fats are an essential part of a healthy diet. The goal is moderation. Be sure to eat a moderate amount of healthy unsaturated fatty acids, especially omega-3s, and avoid saturated and trans fats as much as possible.

Unhealthy types of fats, such as saturated and trans fats, raise your "bad" LDL cholesterol and lower the "good" HDL cholesterol, thereby increasing plaque buildup. Unsaturated fats, such as polyunsaturated omega-3 fatty acids, have been shown to have the opposite effect. These healthy unsaturated fats are found in low concentrations in fruits and vegetables, and in higher concentrations in fish.

## What You Should Eat

Understanding these basic concepts, let's now focus on what's important: FOOD! The DASH diet is all about eating lean protein, complex carbohydrates, and a limited amount of healthy fats, while trying to avoid unhealthy fats, sodium, and simple sugars. To do this, your diet should consist primarily of whole grains, fruits and vegetables, and lean protein and fish. In addition, you should try to avoid sweets, fried and fatty foods, and salty foods.

But instead of fixating on the foods you shouldn't have, let's concentrate on the good stuff. There are worlds of new flavor to be discovered on the DASH diet! By eliminating overly processed, packaged food, and getting back to the basics, you will discover the beauty of real food. Without the cloak of salt and grease, you'll be able to taste the freshness and true flavor of your ingredients. And you'll be amazed by how quick and delicious healthy cooking can be. *The DASH Diet 30-Minute Cookbook* was written with practicality in mind, offering 175 simple recipes that make caring for yourself and your health easy and pleasurable.

## Suggested Servings

The DASH diet takes the guesswork out of healthy eating by offering optimal amounts or "suggested servings" of the foods you should be consuming on a daily basis. The DASH diet suggests the following amounts:

- Whole Grains: 6–8 daily servings
- Lean Meats or Fish: 6 daily servings or fewer
- Vegetables: 4–5 daily servings
- Fruits: 4–5 daily servings
- Lean Dairy Products: 2–3 daily servings
- Fats and Oils: 2–3 daily servings or fewer
- Nuts, Seeds, or Legumes: 4–5 weekly servings
- Sweets and Added Sugars: 5 weekly servings or fewer

These servings vary based on individual caloric needs, but the proportions should stay relatively fixed. For example, if you are very active and burn roughly 3,000 calories per day, you may need to increase whole grains to 9–12 servings, fruits and vegetables to 6–8 servings, and so on. Similarly, if you are sedentary, you may want to proportionally reduce the suggested servings or increase your level of activity.

## Putting It All Together

The biggest challenge of any diet is making the commitment. *The DASH Diet 30-Minute Cookbook* was written with this in mind. The following meal planning section will help guide your successful transition to the DASH diet and provide the long-term confidence you need to stay committed. Here are 5 great tips to get you started.

1. **Stop adding salt to your food.** Added salt is unnecessary, especially when using any type of processed food.
2. **Opt for salt-free spice blends.** Most supermarkets carry an array of salt-free seasonings and you can also make your own (try the terrific Salt-Free Chili Seasoning recipe in Chapter 7). Find a favorite salt-free blend and keep it on hand (or in your purse) always! Invest in

dried herbs and ground spices and store them in a cool, dark place to maintain freshness.

3. **Read labels.** When buying any sort of packaged food, check the nutrition facts carefully. Low-sodium products contain 140 mg per serving or less. Low-fat products contain 3 grams of fat per serving or less.

4. **Pick "Salt-Free," "No-Salt-Added," and "Low-Sodium" products.** Salt-free foods will save you hundreds of milligrams of sodium per serving. Locate salt-free or low-sodium versions of your favorite products and leave the old ones behind.

5. **Before baking, buy these!** Traditional leavening agents contain hundreds of milligrams of sodium. Sodium-free baking powder and baking soda are available in local health food stores and online on Amazon.com, *http://healthyheartmarket.com*, and other retailers.

## Meal Planning: Getting Started

Any diet is easier to maintain when you are well prepared, and the DASH diet is no exception. The recipes in *The DASH Diet 30-Minute Cookbook* require very little time, only standard kitchen equipment, and ingredients that are readily available in most supermarkets. Your DASH diet success is virtually guaranteed! Any specialty products, such as the sodium-free leavening agents just discussed, are noted in the recipes.

Begin your transition by stocking your new DASH kitchen. Think about the ingredients you use on a regular basis and purchase healthier versions of those staples, such as white whole-wheat flour, low-sodium canned goods like tomatoes and beans, and salt-free seasoning. Then take some time to thumb through the recipes in this book, deciding what you would like to make for the next week. Compose a list of what you'll need to grab from the grocery store (or online) to create those meals, and get your kitchen ready so that meal preparation is as simple as possible.

You can also prepare ahead of time by making big batches of your favorite dishes on weekends and freezing them for easy weeknight meals. Many of the recipes in this book include tips for doubling and freezing batches, making this process even easier. That way, you're always prepared when hunger strikes and you're tempted to reach for an unhealthy snack or hop into that drive-thru line. If you're a snacking fiend and can't help indulging in a treat here and there, make sure you get rid of junk food while leaving healthy snacks where you can see them. This can mean buying a bag of unsalted trail mix instead of potato chips, or making an extra batch of Baked Apple Slices (Chapter 6) or Cheesy Seasoned Popcorn (Chapter 5) for when the craving hits. If you surround yourself with healthier options, you're more likely to snag one of those instead of something loaded with sodium and fat.

Another thing to keep in mind is that you want to limit your sodium intake to 2,300 mg per day, or 1,500 mg if adhering to a low-sodium DASH diet. Make sure that the meals you've planned are all within this limit and that you're getting a variety of fruits and vegetables in your diet. Check frozen foods, canned goods, and prepackaged foods carefully for hidden sodium. When selecting products, opt for "no-salt-added" or "reduced sodium" versions. And remember that you also don't need *extra* salt, so forget the shaker and eliminate additional sources of sodium whenever possible. Your healthy choices will add up quickly, lowering your blood pressure and improving health in a myriad of ways.

## What to Buy

When shopping, stick to the outside aisles of the supermarket. Load your cart with fresh fruit and vegetables, lean sources of protein (meat, fish, beans, tofu), low-fat dairy products or nondairy milk, and whole grain bread and pasta. Aim for low-fat, low-cholesterol, low-sodium foods that are high in vitamins and minerals, fiber, and protein. These form the basis of the DASH diet. Focus on unprocessed, whole foods. If the list of ingredients is longer than this paragraph, then don't buy it. The same can be said for foods with extensive packaging or extended expiration dates. Also keep in mind that real food spoils more quickly.

## Get Ready!

Now that you're armed with a better understanding of the DASH diet and how to get started, it's time to dive into dozens of deliciously quick and easy recipes! The remainder of *The DASH Diet 30-Minute Cookbook* will guide you through each step as you make hearty breakfast dishes, wholesome dinners, and even mouthwatering desserts. Congratulations on taking the first step in your DASH diet journey—get ready for a happier, healthier you!

# CHAPTER 2

Breakfasts

Homemade Sausage Patties

Maple Turkey Sausage

Baking Powder Biscuits

Scrambled Eggs with Apples,
    Sage, and Swiss Cheese

Sweet Corn Muffins

Diner-Style Home Fries

Saturday Morning Pancakes

Chocolate Pancakes

Orange Cornmeal Pancakes

Instant Banana Oatmeal

Brown Sugar Cinnamon Oatmeal

Hot Honey Porridge

Homemade Granola

Hearty Tofu Scramble with
    Spinach, Mushrooms,
    and Peppers

Swiss Cheese Mini Quiches

Oven-Baked Apple Pancake

Sunday Morning Waffles

Pumpkin Waffles

Banana Nut Muffins

Coffee Cake Muffins

# Homemade Sausage Patties

**Prep Time:** 5 minutes
**Cook Time:** 10 minutes
**Total Time:** 15 minutes
**Serves 8**

## INGREDIENTS

2 pounds lean ground pork

1 egg white

2 teaspoons brown sugar

2½ teaspoons ground sage

1 teaspoon dried marjoram

¾ teaspoon dried red pepper flakes

½ teaspoon freshly ground black pepper

¼ teaspoon ground rosemary

Welcome back to breakfast, low-sodium dieters! These delicious homemade sausage patties are scented with sage and have a nice red pepper kick. But sausage isn't just for breakfast. It makes a terrific topping for pizza, adds spice and interest to plain pasta and sauce, and elevates boring meatloaf to something special. Double the batch whenever you make this dish, and freeze leftover patties for use in future recipes. Steps like this will save you time, and make following the DASH diet easier and tastier!

1. Combine ingredients in a large bowl and mix well using a fork or your hands. Form mixture into 16 (roughly) 2-inch patties.

2. Heat griddle or skillet over medium heat and brown patties on both sides, about 5 minutes per side. Lower heat to medium-low or low if they seem to be burning. Drain on paper towels before serving.

**Per Serving (2 patties)**
Calories: 186
Fat: 9 grams
Protein: 22 grams
Sodium: 67 milligrams

Fiber: 0 grams
Carbohydrates: 1 gram
Sugar: 1 gram

# Maple Turkey Sausage

**Prep Time:** 5 minutes
**Cook Time:** 8 minutes
**Total Time:** 13 minutes
**Serves 8**

## INGREDIENTS

2 pounds lean ground turkey

1 egg white

1 tablespoon pure maple syrup

1 tablespoon ground sage

½ teaspoon dried red pepper flakes

½ teaspoon fennel seed

½ teaspoon freshly ground black pepper

½ teaspoon ground rosemary

¼ teaspoon garlic powder

Perfect for those avoiding pork or simply looking for another lean breakfast meat. These homemade patties are super speedy, subtly sweet, and absolutely delicious. Feel free to substitute lean ground chicken for the turkey. For another twist on the recipe, instead of forming into patties, brown the mixture along with chopped onion, garlic, and apple, and serve with scrambled eggs for a hearty breakfast bowl.

1. Combine ingredients in a large bowl and mix well using a fork or your hands. The mixture will be sticky. Form into 16 (roughly) 2-inch patties.

2. Heat griddle or skillet over medium and brown patties on both sides, about 4 minutes per side. Lower heat to medium-low or low if they seem to be burning. Drain on paper towels before serving.

**Per Serving (2 patties)**

Calories: 161

Fat: 7 grams

Protein: 22 grams

Sodium: 87 milligrams

Fiber: 0 grams

Carbohydrates: 1 gram

Sugar: 1 gram

# Baking Powder Biscuits

**Prep Time:** 5 minutes
**Cook Time:** 10 minutes
**Total Time:** 15 minutes
**Yields 1 dozen**

## INGREDIENTS

1 cup unbleached all-purpose flour
1 cup white whole-wheat flour
1 tablespoon sugar
4 teaspoons sodium-free baking powder
4 tablespoons non-hydrogenated vegetable shortening (e.g., Spectrum Naturals)
1 egg white
⅔ cup low-fat milk

These light, flaky biscuits are table ready in 15 minutes, making them a great choice for breakfast or any meal. Instead of traditional vegetable shortening, this recipe uses non-hydrogenated shortening. Non-hydrogenated vegetable shortening is made naturally from pressed oils that are solid at room temperature. It's also free of trans fats and cholesterol, making it a good alternative to butter when baking. Spectrum Naturals Organic All Vegetable Shortening is sold at Whole Foods markets and online. If you don't have some on hand, you can substitute unsalted butter for the shortening.

1. Preheat oven to 450°F. Take out a baking sheet and set aside.

2. Place the flours, sugar, and baking powder into a mixing bowl and whisk well to combine.

3. Cut the shortening into the mixture using your fingers, and work until it resembles coarse crumbs. Add the egg white and milk and stir to combine.

4. Turn the dough out onto a lightly floured surface and knead 1 minute. Roll dough to (roughly) ¾-inch thickness and cut into 12 (2-inch) rounds.

5. Place rounds on the baking sheet. Place baking sheet on middle rack in oven and bake 10 minutes.

6. Remove baking sheet and place biscuits on a wire rack to cool.

**Per Serving (1 biscuit)**
Calories: 118
Fat: 4 grams
Protein: 3 grams
Sodium: 13 milligrams

Fiber: 1 gram
Carbohydrates: 16 grams
Sugar: <1 gram

# Scrambled Eggs with Apples, Sage, and Swiss Cheese

**Prep Time:** 2 minutes
**Cook Time:** 8 minutes
**Total Time:** 10 minutes
**Serves 2**

## INGREDIENTS

2 large eggs
1 medium apple, chopped
1 shallot, chopped
¼ cup shredded Swiss cheese
1 teaspoon chopped fresh sage (or ½ tea-spoon dried sage)
Freshly ground black pepper, to taste

This spectacular combination of tastes and textures seems tailor-made for fall. The warmth and softness of the eggs, the tang of the Swiss, the play of apple against shallot, and the sage—don't forget the sage! That woodsy scent draws everything together. When it comes to cheese, Swiss is always a safe bet for those on the DASH diet. Not only is it often lower in sodium than other cheeses, but some brands even offer salt-free varieties. If you can't find pre-shredded Swiss, just slice or shred it yourself.

1. Break eggs into a small bowl and beat well; set aside.

2. Place a nonstick skillet over medium-low heat. Add the chopped apple and shallot and cook, stirring, until soft but not brown, roughly 3–5 minutes.

3. Add the beaten eggs. Let set roughly 30 seconds, then, stirring, cook additional 30 seconds to 1 minute, until egg is almost cooked. Add Swiss cheese and stir.

4. Remove from heat and serve immediately, sprinkling with sage and freshly ground black pepper.

**Per Serving (1 cup)**
Calories: 165
Fat: 8 grams
Protein: 10 grams
Sodium: 97 milligrams
Fiber: 2 grams
Carbohydrates: 12 grams
Sugar: 8 grams

# Sweet Corn Muffins

**Prep Time:** 5 minutes
**Cook Time:** 15 minutes
**Total Time:** 20 minutes
**Yields 1 dozen**

## INGREDIENTS

1 cup cornmeal

1 cup white whole-wheat flour

½ cup sugar

1 tablespoon sodium-free baking powder

¾ cup nondairy milk

½ cup canola oil

1 teaspoon pure vanilla extract

**Sodium-Free Baking Powder**
Standard baking powder, the kind typically sold in supermarkets, contains hundreds of milligrams of sodium per serving, and is not recommended on the DASH diet. Two brands of sodium-free baking powder are available and achieve the same great rise in baked goods: Ener-G Baking Powder can be purchased online; Hain Pure Foods Featherweight Baking Powder is sold online, at Whole Foods markets, and other select stores.

They're sweet, they're soft, and they're even a little crunchy up top. These cholesterol-free muffins are amazing, and make any breakfast, lunch, or dinner better. Best of all? They're table-ready in just 20 minutes! For extra nutrition, add a tablespoon of ground flaxseed to the batter, along with a few tablespoons of water. Ground flaxseed is sold at most supermarkets, and is a great source of heart-healthy omega-3s.

1. Preheat the oven to 400°F. Line a 12-muffin tin with paper liners and set aside.

2. Place the cornmeal, flour, sugar, and baking powder into a mixing bowl and whisk well to combine.

3. Add the nondairy milk, oil, and vanilla and stir just until combined.

4. Divide the batter evenly between the muffin cups. Place muffin tin on middle rack in oven and bake for 15 minutes.

5. Remove from oven and place on a wire rack to cool.

**Per Serving (1 muffin)**

| | |
|---|---|
| Calories: 203 | Fiber: 2 grams |
| Fat: 9 grams | Carbohydrates: 26 grams |
| Protein: 3 grams | Sugar: 9 grams |
| Sodium: 11 milligrams | |

# Diner-Style Home Fries

**Prep Time:** 10 minutes
**Cook Time:** 17 minutes
**Total Time:** 27 minutes
**Serves 6**

## INGREDIENTS

4 medium potatoes, cut into ½-inch cubes

1 teaspoon olive oil

1 medium onion, diced

1 medium sweet bell pepper, diced

1 tablespoon salt-free tomato paste

2 teaspoons ground sweet paprika

½ teaspoon dried thyme

½ teaspoon garlic powder

½ teaspoon ground rosemary

¼ teaspoon freshly ground black pepper

Tender, seasoned potatoes sautéed with onion and bell pepper make a magnificent side dish at breakfast; reheat and enjoy leftovers later in the day! Home fries and hashes can be crafted using almost anything. Instead of standard russets, try sweet potatoes. Dice leftover meat, hard-boiled eggs, or low-sodium Swiss cheese and add to the mix. Or chop up a wide variety of vegetables and make yourself a super vegan hash. To save time and money, substitute pre-cut frozen veggies, like onions and peppers, for fresh.

1. Place diced potatoes into a microwave-safe bowl and cover with plastic wrap. Microwave for 7 minutes.

2. While potatoes are cooking, heat oil in a nonstick skillet over medium heat. Add onion and bell pepper and cook, stirring, for 7 minutes.

3. Add cooked potatoes to skillet, along with tomato paste and seasonings. Stir to combine, then cook, stirring, another 2–3 minutes. Remove from heat and serve.

**Per Serving (1 cup)**
Calories: 101
Fat: 1 gram
Protein: 2 grams
Sodium: 10 milligrams

Fiber: 2 grams
Carbohydrates: 21 grams
Sugar: 2 grams

# Saturday Morning Pancakes

**Prep Time:** 5 minutes
**Cook Time:** 7 minutes per pancake
**Total Time:** 12 minutes
**Serves 4**

## INGREDIENTS

1⅓ cups white whole-wheat flour

¼ cup sugar

1 tablespoon sodium-free baking powder

1½ cups low-fat milk

1 egg white

1 tablespoon canola oil

1 tablespoon pure vanilla extract

Weekends were made for hot, fluffy pancakes. This tried-and-true recipe is great with any type of flour, and can be adapted for vegans by using nondairy milk and egg replacement powder. To save yourself hunger and hassle on weekdays, double pancake or waffle recipes on weekends, then place leftovers between small sheets of waxed paper and store in plastic bags in the freezer. A frozen pancake or waffle will defrost in minutes, providing a quick and easy breakfast anytime.

1. Measure the flour, sugar, and baking powder into a mixing bowl and whisk well to combine.

2. Add the milk, egg white, oil, and vanilla. Mix well and let sit for 1–2 minutes to thicken.

3. Place nonstick griddle or skillet on stove and turn heat to medium-low. Pour batter onto heated griddle. When pancake has bubbled on top and is nicely browned on bottom (approximately 2–4 minutes), flip over. Brown on second side another 2–3 minutes. If pancakes are browning too quickly, lower heat to low.

4. Repeat process with remaining batter. Serve pancakes warm.

**Per Serving (2 (4-inch) pancakes)**

| | |
|---|---|
| Calories: 266 | |
| Fat: 5 grams | Fiber: 4 grams |
| Protein: 9 grams | Carbohydrates: 46 grams |
| Sodium: 56 milligrams | Sugar: 17 grams |

# Chocolate Pancakes

**Prep Time:** 5 minutes
**Cook Time:** 7 minutes per pancake
**Total Time:** 12 minutes
**Serves 4**

## INGREDIENTS

1 cup white whole-wheat flour

¼ cup unsweetened cocoa powder

¼ cup sugar

1 tablespoon sodium-free baking powder

1½ cups low-fat milk

1 large egg

2 tablespoons canola oil

½ teaspoon pure vanilla extract

### From Soup to . . . Pancakes?

Soup ladles aren't just for soup. They work wonderfully for measuring and pouring pancake batter onto any hot cooking surface. The resulting pancakes will be perfectly shaped and sized, and you'll never worry about messy cleanup! Ladles also work wonderfully when measuring waffle batter.

Did you know it takes just twelve minutes to create a completely decadent, yet totally guilt-free breakfast? It's true! Make any morning feel like a special occasion. Add chocolate chips, dried cranberries, or chopped nuts to the batter for an extra-special treat. Or for different flavors, experiment with spices such as ground cinnamon or cardamom.

1. Measure the flour, cocoa powder, sugar, and baking powder into a mixing bowl and whisk well to combine.

2. Add the milk, egg, oil, and vanilla. Mix well.

3. Place nonstick griddle or skillet on stove and turn heat to medium-low. Pour batter onto heated griddle. When pancake has bubbled on top and is nicely browned on bottom (approximately 2–4 minutes), flip over. Brown on second side another 2–3 minutes. If pancakes are browning too quickly, lower heat to low.

4. Repeat process with remaining batter. Serve pancakes warm, with whipped cream and real maple syrup if desired.

**Per Serving (2 (4-inch) pancakes)**

| | |
|---|---|
| Calories: 251 | Fiber: 5 grams |
| Fat: 7 grams | Carbohydrates: 42 grams |
| Protein: 9 grams | Sugar: 17 grams |
| Sodium: 60 milligrams | |

# Orange Cornmeal Pancakes

**Prep Time:** 5 minutes
**Cook Time:** 7 minutes per pancake
**Total Time:** 12 minutes
**Serves 4**

## INGREDIENTS

⅔ cup white whole-wheat flour

⅔ cup cornmeal

1 tablespoon sodium-free baking powder

¼ cup sugar

3 tablespoons freshly squeezed orange juice

1½ teaspoons minced orange zest

1 cup low-fat milk

1 egg white

Wake up with bright citrus flavor and a sweet corn crunch. These light, fluffy pancakes are so good, you may even pass on the syrup. Pressed for time? Try wrapping a pancake around a ripe banana, burrito-style, for a quick breakfast on the go—no knife and fork necessary!

1. Measure all the ingredients into a mixing bowl and stir well to combine.

2. Place nonstick griddle or skillet on stove and turn heat to medium-low. Pour batter onto heated griddle. When pancake has bubbled on top and is nicely browned on bottom (approximately 2–4 minutes) flip over. Brown on second side another 2–3 minutes. If pancakes are browning too quickly, lower heat to low.

3. Repeat process with remaining batter. Serve immediately.

**Per Serving (2 (4-inch) pancakes)**

| | |
|---|---|
| Calories: 223 | |
| Fat: 2 grams | Fiber: 4 grams |
| Protein: 7 grams | Carbohydrates: 46 grams |
| Sodium: 48 milligrams | Sugar: 16 grams |

# Instant Banana Oatmeal

**Prep Time:** 1 minute
**Cook Time:** 2 minutes
**Total Time:** 3 minutes
**Serves 1**

## INGREDIENTS

½ cup quick oats

½ cup water

1 ripe banana, mashed

### Differences in Oats

Oats come in three main types. Quick or instant oats have been precooked and dried. They have the fastest cooking time and are great for making oatmeal or adding to baked goods. Old-fashioned rolled oats have been put through a steaming process to speed cooking. They're considered all-purpose and work well in most recipes. Steel-cut oats are cut, not rolled. They have a chewy texture that's good for oatmeal and other recipes, but because of their longer cooking time, aren't ideal for everything.

Say hello to your new breakfast buddy! With just 3 ingredients and 3 minutes of your time, you'll have a meal that'll keep you full and satisfied all morning long. Not only is this all-natural recipe low in sodium, but it's also low-fat, gluten-free, cholesterol-free, free of refined sugar and salt, high in fiber, and absolutely delicious.

1. Measure the oats and water into a microwave-safe bowl and stir to combine.

2. Place bowl in microwave and heat on high for 2 minutes.

3. Remove bowl from microwave and stir in the mashed banana. Enjoy as is or sprinkle with a dash of ground cinnamon.

**Per Serving (1⅓ cups)**

| | | | |
|---|---|---|---|
| Calories: 243 | | Fiber: 6 grams | |
| Fat: 3 grams | | Carbohydrates: 50 grams | |
| Protein: 6 grams | | Sugar: 12 grams | |
| Sodium: 6 milligrams | | | |

# Brown Sugar Cinnamon Oatmeal

**Prep Time:** 1 minute
**Cook Time:** 4 minutes
**Total Time:** 5 minutes
**Serves 4**

## INGREDIENTS

2 cups low-fat milk

1½ teaspoons pure vanilla extract

1⅓ cups quick oats

¼ cup light brown sugar

½ teaspoon ground cinnamon

I created this recipe especially for my daughters, who love those flavored instant oatmeal packets you can buy at the store. This recipe produces a creamy oatmeal every bit as delicious as those instant packets, but without the high sodium and artificial flavors. And it's just as quick! Five minutes from start to finish and breakfast is done.

1. Measure the milk and vanilla into a medium saucepan and bring to a boil over medium-high heat.

2. Once boiling, reduce heat to medium. Stir in oats, brown sugar, and cinnamon, and cook, stirring, 2–3 minutes.

3. Serve immediately, sprinkled with additional cinnamon if desired.

**Per Serving (⅔ cup)**
Calories: 208
Fat: 3 grams
Protein: 8 grams
Sodium: 58 milligrams

Fiber: 2 grams
Carbohydrates: 38 grams
Sugar: 20 grams

# Hot Honey Porridge

**Prep Time:** 5 minutes
**Cook Time:** 10 minutes
**Total Time:** 15 minutes
**Serves 4**

## INGREDIENTS

¾ cup bulgur wheat
½ cup rolled oats
3 cups boiling water
¼ cup honey

A warm and filling alternative to oatmeal, this healthy multigrain cereal has a soft honey taste and a creamy, slightly chewy texture. For variety, add raisins, chopped nuts, or a dash of cinnamon to the mix. Bulgur is a whole wheat grain that has been cracked and partially precooked. It's naturally vegan, low-calorie, low-fat, and high in fiber. It can also be incorporated into many dishes as a substitute for rice, couscous, barley, or quinoa.

1. Place the bulgur wheat and rolled oats into a saucepan. Add the boiling water and stir to combine.

2. Place pan over high heat and bring to a boil. Once boiling, reduce heat to low, then cover and simmer for 10 minutes, stirring occasionally.

3. Remove from heat, stir in honey, and serve immediately.

**Per Serving (½ cup)**

| | |
|---|---|
| Calories: 172 | Fiber: 5 grams |
| Fat: 1 gram | Carbohydrates: 40 grams |
| Protein: 4 grams | Sugar: 17 grams |
| Sodium: 5 milligrams | |

# Homemade Granola

**Prep Time:** 5 minutes
**Cook Time:** 25 minutes
**Total Time:** 30 minutes
**Yields 10 cups**

## INGREDIENTS

6 cups quick or old-fashioned oats

1¼ cups unsalted chopped nuts (your choice)

½ cup dried unsweetened coconut (shredded)

1 teaspoon ground cinnamon

½ teaspoon ground ginger

¼ teaspoon ground cloves

¼ teaspoon ground nutmeg

1 cup pure maple syrup

1½ tablespoons pure vanilla extract

2 cups chopped dried fruit (your choice)

### Cereal Makes a Great Snack, Too!

Most breakfast foods are fast, making them a great choice for quick meals or between-meal snacks. Topped with fresh fruit, like bananas or berries, and low-fat milk, granola will satisfy a craving for sweets while keeping you healthy and well. You can layer it with low-fat yogurt and fresh fruit for healthy parfaits, or mix in some chocolate chips and unsalted nuts for a high-energy trail mix.

Commercial breakfast cereals often contain large quantities of sodium. Get around this is by making your own. Subtly sweet and super crunchy, this granola keeps well for weeks when stored in an airtight container. The dried fruit is stirred in after the cereal has fully cooled, so it stays soft. Unsweetened shredded coconut lends a lot of flavor without much sodium, but you can omit it if you're also watching your fat intake.

1. Preheat oven to 350°F. Take out 2 baking sheets, spray lightly with oil, and set aside.

2. In a large mixing bowl, combine the oats, chopped nuts, shredded coconut, cinnamon, ginger, cloves, and nutmeg.

3. Add the maple syrup and vanilla, and stir until everything is thoroughly coated.

4. Divide the mixture between the 2 baking sheets. Place sheets on middle rack in oven and bake until golden brown, roughly 25 minutes. Two or three times during baking, remove sheets and carefully stir contents before returning to oven. This will ensure even baking so the granola does not burn.

5. Once golden brown, remove baking sheets from oven and set aside to cool fully. Once cooled, stir the dried fruit into the mixture. Store in an airtight container.

**Per Serving (1 cup)**
Calories: 266
Fat: 10 grams
Protein: 5 grams
Sodium: 7 milligrams

Fiber: 4 grams
Carbohydrates: 42 grams
Sugar: 19 grams

# Hearty Tofu Scramble with Spinach, Mushrooms, and Peppers

Prep Time: 5 minutes
Cook Time: 10 minutes
Total Time: 15 minutes
Serves 4

## INGREDIENTS

1 medium onion, diced

2 cloves garlic, minced

8 ounces sliced mushrooms

1 medium bell pepper, diced

6 ounces fresh baby spinach

1 pound firm or extra-firm tofu, drained

3 tablespoons nutritional yeast flakes

1 tablespoon low-sodium soy sauce

1½ teaspoons all-purpose salt-free seasoning

¼ teaspoon freshly ground black pepper, or to taste

### Nutritional Yeast Flakes

Nutritional yeast is a type of inactive yeast with a zingy, cheese-like flavor, making it a great substitute for cheese in low-sodium and vegan diets. The little yellow flakes can be sprinkled on popcorn, pasta, or anything you'd like to perk up. Nutritional yeast also contains important vitamins such as vitamin $B_{12}$, often found in meat, making it an especially nutritious supplement for vegetarians and vegans. To save time and money, buy it in bulk and store it in an airtight container in the freezer.

Sautéed veggies and yummy seasoning make tofu a tasty cholesterol-free stand-in for scrambled eggs. And for those unfamiliar with nutritional yeast, get ready to be amazed! Nutritional yeast is a type of inactive yeast with fabulous cheese-like flavor and a mere 11 mg of sodium per tablespoon! Find it at supermarkets, natural food stores, and online.

1. Place a nonstick skillet over medium heat. Add the onion, garlic, mushrooms, and bell pepper and cook, stirring, for 5 minutes.

2. Add the spinach to the pan, then crumble the tofu over top, keeping it in rather large chunks. Add the nutritional yeast, soy sauce, salt-free seasoning, and black pepper. Let the mixture cook another 5 minutes, stirring to combine as the spinach begins to wilt.

3. Remove from heat and serve immediately.

**Per Serving (1½ cups)**

Calories: 156

Fat: 6 grams

Protein: 16 grams

Sodium: 176 milligrams

Fiber: 4 grams

Carbohydrates: 10 grams

Sugar: 3 grams

# Swiss Cheese Mini Quiches

**Prep Time:** 5 minutes
**Cook Time:** 25 minutes
**Total Time:** 30 minutes
**Yields 1 dozen**

## INGREDIENTS

¾ cup plus 2 tablespoons unbleached all-purpose flour, divided
½ teaspoon salt-free all-purpose seasoning
¼ teaspoon dried dill
2 tablespoons unsalted butter
Cold water, as needed

### FILLING

2 large eggs
⅔ cup low-fat milk
⅓ cup nonfat or low-fat sour cream
6 tablespoons shredded Swiss cheese
¼ cup chopped fresh chives or green onion
Freshly ground black pepper, to taste

These tasty treats look impressive, but require very little preparation and equipment—all you need is a rolling pin, muffin tin, and 30 minutes! For even faster quiches, make the dough ahead of time and freeze. Place the rounds onto a parchment-lined baking sheet, freeze 20–30 minutes, then transfer to an airtight container. Double or even triple the batch of dough, and you'll have ready-made crusts whenever the urge strikes. Feel free to alter the filling ingredients and seasonings to suit your taste. Add sautéed mushrooms, onion, and spinach (cooked and well-drained) or try low-sodium bacon with jalapeños. The possibilities are endless.

1. Preheat oven to 350°F. Take out a 12-muffin tin and set aside.

2. To make the crust, measure ¾ cup flour, all-purpose seasoning, and dill into a mixing bowl and whisk to combine. Cut the butter into the mixture using your hands, working it until a fine crumb has been achieved.

3. Add cold water, ½ tablespoon at a time, until the dough just comes together. Roll the dough out thinly and cut into 12 roughly 2-inch circles using a biscuit cutter or drinking glass. Lightly spray the muffin tin with oil and line each cup with a round of dough.

4. To prepare the filling, beat the eggs, milk, sour cream, and 2 tablespoons flour in a mixing bowl until well combined.

5. Divide mixture evenly between the muffin tin cups. Top each with ½ tablespoon shredded Swiss

continued on next page

cheese and 1 teaspoon of fresh chives. Sprinkle with freshly ground black pepper, to taste.

6. Place tin on middle rack in oven and bake for 25 minutes. Remove from oven and let rest for a few minutes. Remove mini quiches by sliding a knife around edges and gently lifting up. Serve warm or at room temperature.

**Per Serving (2 mini quiches)**
Calories: 170
Fat: 7 grams
Protein: 7 grams
Sodium: 93 milligrams

Fiber: 1 gram
Carbohydrates: 18 grams
Sugar: 2 grams

# Oven-Baked Apple Pancake

**Prep Time:** 5 minutes
**Cook Time:** 25 minutes
**Total Time:** 30 minutes
**Serves 8**

## INGREDIENTS

2 cups diced apple

1 tablespoon pure vanilla extract

1 tablespoon sodium-free baking powder

1 cup unbleached all-purpose flour

⅓ cup unsweetened applesauce

⅓ cup real maple syrup

¾ cup nondairy milk

1 tablespoon sugar

½ teaspoon ground cinnamon

A light and fluffy pancake made without milk and eggs? It's true! Moist, airy, and delicious, this cholesterol-free pancake will impress with its taste and simplicity. The oven does all the work: Just whisk together the ingredients, pour, and bake. In just 30 minutes, you've got a healthy, heavenly way to fill your belly.

1. Preheat oven to 400°F. Lightly spray a large oven-proof skillet with oil.

2. Place the apple, vanilla, baking powder, flour, applesauce, maple syrup, and nondairy milk into a large mixing bowl and whisk well to combine. Pour batter into the prepared skillet and smooth top to even.

3. Combine the sugar and cinnamon in a small bowl and sprinkle evenly over the batter.

4. Place skillet on middle rack in oven and bake for 25 minutes. Remove from oven. Carefully loosen pancake from skillet using a spatula. Slice like a pizza into 8 pieces and serve immediately.

**Per Serving (1 slice)**
Calories: 126
Fat: 1 gram
Protein: 2 grams
Sodium: 10 milligrams

Fiber: 1 gram
Carbohydrates: 27 grams
Sugar: 13 grams

# Sunday Morning Waffles

**Prep Time:** 5 minutes
**Cook Time:** 5 minutes per waffle
**Total Time:** 10 minutes
**Serves 6**

## INGREDIENTS

1⅔ cups unbleached all-purpose flour

¼ cup sugar

1 tablespoon sodium-free baking powder

1½ cups low-fat milk

2 teaspoons pure vanilla extract

2 tablespoons canola oil

2 egg whites

### Waffle Tip

To keep waffles warm while you finish making the entire batch, place cooked waffles directly on the middle rack of a preheated 200°F oven. Once all are made, remove waffles from oven and serve. When serving, *do not stack* the waffles. The moisture from the waffles will condense and cause them to go limp and soggy. Always serve waffles in a single layer to keep them fresh and crisp.

Waffles never fail to impress, yet they're so simple to make. As a bonus, they freeze beautifully, so if you double or even triple the batch, you can package, freeze, and then toast for quick weekday breakfasts. For a super-decadent dessert, top homemade waffles with low-fat ice cream, whipped cream, and sprinkles. Don't forget the (unsweetened) cherry on top!

1. Spray waffle iron lightly with oil and preheat. Measure the flour, sugar, and baking powder into a mixing bowl and whisk well to combine. Add milk, vanilla, and canola oil to the dry ingredients and mix well. Let rest for 1–2 minutes to thicken.

2. While batter is thickening, place egg whites into another mixing bowl and beat until they form stiff peaks. Once beaten, gently fold whites into the batter.

3. Ladle batter onto hot surface of waffle iron, being careful to avoid the edges (batter will spread once appliance is closed). Close waffle iron and bake until golden brown, roughly 4–5 minutes.

4. Remove baked waffle from iron and repeat process with remaining batter, re-oiling waffle iron as necessary. Serve immediately.

**Per Serving (1 waffle)**
Calories: 220
Fat: 6 grams
Protein: 7 grams
Sodium: 46 milligrams

Fiber: 4 grams
Carbohydrates: 35 grams
Sugar: 11 grams

# Pumpkin Waffles

**Prep Time:** 7 minutes
**Cook Time:** 18 minutes
**Total Time:** 25 minutes
**Serves 6**

## INGREDIENTS

1 cup pumpkin purée

1 cup white whole-wheat flour

½ cup unbleached all-purpose flour

⅓ cup brown sugar

1½ cups low-fat milk

1 egg white

1 tablespoon canola oil

1 tablespoon sodium-free baking powder

1 tablespoon pure vanilla extract

2 teaspoons ground cinnamon

¼ teaspoon ground allspice

¼ teaspoon ground ginger

Everything's better with pumpkin! Not only does it lend superb color and flavor to any dish, but when carved, it's pure FUN! This low-fat breakfast is packed with healthy whole grains and vitamin A. Top waffles with pure maple syrup for the ultimate taste of fall in New England, any time of year. No carving necessary.

1. Spray waffle iron lightly with oil and preheat. Measure all ingredients into a large mixing bowl and beat until smooth.

2. Ladle batter onto hot surface of waffle iron, being careful to avoid the edges (batter will spread once appliance is closed). Close waffle iron and bake until golden brown, roughly 4–5 minutes.

3. Remove baked waffle from iron and repeat process with remaining batter, re-oiling waffle iron as necessary. Serve immediately.

**Per Serving (1 waffle)**

| | |
|---|---|
| Calories: 219 | Fiber: 4 grams |
| Fat: 3 grams | Carbohydrates: 41 grams |
| Protein: 7 grams | Sugar: 16 grams |
| Sodium: 43 grams | |

# Banana Nut Muffins

**Prep Time:** 5 minutes
**Cook Time:** 18 minutes
**Total Time:** 23 minutes
**Yields 1 dozen**

## INGREDIENTS

1 cup mashed banana

½ cup brown sugar

1 egg white

2 tablespoons canola oil

2 teaspoons pure vanilla extract

½ teaspoon ground cinnamon

2 teaspoons sodium-free baking powder

1½ cups white whole-wheat flour

1 tablespoon low-fat milk

¼ cup chopped walnuts

### Baking with Bananas

Overripe bananas may not look appealing, but they lend fabulous flavor and enhanced sweetness to baked goods and smoothies, and may even eliminate the need for added sugar and oil. If you have overripe bananas on hand and don't have time to bake, seal them in an airtight container and freeze for later use. Once frozen, the banana peels turn deep black, but the flesh inside remains perfectly fine and keeps for months. Feel free to peel them before freezing to make life even easier!

Sweet and moist with great banana flavor, the quintessential muffin gets a whole-grain makeover. This is a wonderful way to use up those overripe spotted bananas sitting on your kitchen counter (and if they're not spotted yet, they will be soon). Add chocolate chips or dried fruit for added fun and flavor.

1. Preheat oven to 375°F. Line a 12-muffin tin with paper liners and set aside.

2. In a mixing bowl, beat together the banana, brown sugar, egg white, oil, vanilla, and cinnamon.

3. Add the baking powder and stir well to combine. Gradually add in the flour, then the milk and walnuts. Stir until everything is incorporated.

4. Spoon batter into muffin cups, filling each roughly ⅔ full. Place tin on middle rack in oven and bake for 18 minutes. Remove from oven and place on wire rack to cool.

**Per Serving (1 muffin)**

Calories: 143

Fat: 4 grams

Protein: 3 grams

Sodium: 9 milligrams

Fiber: 2 grams

Carbohydrates: 25 grams

Sugar: 16 grams

# Coffee Cake Muffins

**Prep Time:** 7 minutes
**Cook Time:** 18 minutes
**Total Time:** 25 minutes
**Yields 1 dozen**

## INGREDIENTS

¼ cup brown sugar

3 tablespoons white whole-wheat flour

½ teaspoon ground cinnamon

5 tablespoons unsalted butter, divided

⅔ cup sugar

½ cup low-fat vanilla yogurt

1 egg white

1 teaspoon pure vanilla extract

2 teaspoons sodium-free baking powder

½ teaspoon sodium-free baking soda

1½ cups unbleached all-purpose flour

2 tablespoons low-fat milk

### Sodium-Free Baking Soda

Standard baking soda contains over 1,200 milligrams of sodium per teaspoon, and is not recommended for those on a DASH diet. Ener-G Baking Soda Substitute is an effective replacement for standard baking soda. In addition to being sodium-free, it's also free of aluminum and gluten, but is high in calcium. Ener-G Baking Soda Substitute is sold online.

Craving crumb-topped coffee cake for breakfast? Bake it up—fast! These muffins have all the moist cinnamon-flecked flavor you've been dreaming of, in half the time. Want to try something new? Swap the low-fat vanilla yogurt for a different flavor (blueberry, chocolate, etc.) and add some chopped fresh fruit, nuts, or chocolate chips.

1. Preheat oven to 350°F. Line a 12-muffin tin with paper liners and set aside.

2. To make the crumb topping, in a small bowl mix together the brown sugar, 3 tablespoons whole-wheat flour, and ground cinnamon. Cut 1 tablespoon butter into the mixture until it becomes crumbly. Set aside.

3. In a mixing bowl, beat the remaining 4 tablespoons butter with the sugar. Add the yogurt, egg white, and vanilla, and mix until smooth.

4. Add the baking powder and baking soda, then gradually add in the all-purpose flour. Stir in the milk.

5. Divide the batter evenly between the muffin cups. Sprinkle the crumb topping evenly over the batter.

6. Place tin on middle rack in oven and bake for 18–20 minutes. Remove from oven and set on wire rack to cool.

**Per Serving (1 muffin)**

| | |
|---|---|
| Calories: 176 | Fiber: 1 gram |
| Fat: 5 grams | Carbohydrates: 29 grams |
| Protein: 3 grams | Sugar: 15 grams |
| Sodium: 13 milligrams | |

# CHAPTER 3

# Salads and Dressings

Sweet Potato Salad with
  Maple Vinaigrette

Warm Potato Salad with Spinach

Garlic Potato Salad

Veggie Pasta Salad with
  Zesty Italian Dressing

Edamame Salad with Corn
  and Cranberries

The Best 3-Bean Salad *Ever*!

Creamy Low-Sodium Coleslaw

Salt-Free Mayonnaise

Southwestern Beet Slaw

Simple Autumn Salad

Summer Corn Salad with
  Peppers and Avocado

Curried Tofu Salad

Tart Apple Salad with Honey
  Yogurt Dressing

Whole-Wheat Couscous Salad
  with Citrus and Cilantro

Tomato, Cucumber,
  and Basil Salad

Tropical Chicken Salad

Lemon Vinaigrette

Sesame Ginger Vinaigrette

Tomato Garlic Dressing

Apple Honey Mustard Vinaigrette

# Sweet Potato Salad with Maple Vinaigrette

**Prep Time:** 10 minutes
**Cook Time:** 20 minutes
**Total Time:** 30 minutes
**Serves 6**

## INGREDIENTS

4 small/medium sweet potatoes
1 (15-ounce) can no-salt-added garbanzo beans
4 scallions, sliced
1 shallot, minced
2 tablespoons pure maple syrup
2 tablespoons freshly squeezed lemon juice
1½ teaspoons olive oil
½ teaspoon dry ground mustard
¼ teaspoon freshly ground black pepper

In one word: *Yum!* This hearty salad makes a healthy and filling one-dish meal. For more color, add a small handful of dried cranberries. For a spicier version, substitute black beans for the garbanzos, add minced garlic instead of shallot, omit the mustard, and swap lime juice for the lemon. Then add a teaspoon of ground cumin and another of salt-free chili seasoning. Stir in a handful of chopped fresh cilantro and serve!

1. Place unpeeled sweet potatoes into a pot and add enough water to cover by a couple of inches. Bring to a boil over high heat. Once boiling, reduce heat to medium-high and simmer until tender, about 20 minutes.

2. Remove pot from heat and drain. Place the sweet potatoes under cold running water until cool enough to handle, then peel and cut into 1-inch chunks.

3. Place sweet potatoes into a mixing bowl, along with the beans, scallions, and shallot.

4. In a small bowl, whisk together the remaining ingredients and then pour over salad. Toss gently to coat.

5. Serve immediately or cover and refrigerate until ready to serve.

**Per Serving (1 cup)**
Calories: 224
Fat: 3 grams
Protein: 7 grams
Sodium: 33 milligrams
Fiber: 8 grams
Carbohydrates: 42 grams
Sugar: 13 grams

# Warm Potato Salad with Spinach

Prep Time: 10 minutes
Cook Time: 15 minutes
Total Time: 25 minutes
Serves 8

## INGREDIENTS

3 pounds small new potatoes or fingerlings

4 cups fresh baby spinach

5 tablespoons red wine vinegar

5 tablespoons olive oil

2 tablespoons water

1 tablespoon no-salt-added prepared mustard

1 tablespoon agave nectar

1 teaspoon garlic powder

1 teaspoon all-purpose salt-free seasoning

½ teaspoon dried dill

½ teaspoon dried Italian seasoning

½ teaspoon dried thyme

Freshly ground black pepper, to taste

### What Is Agave Nectar?

Agave nectar is a liquid sweetener derived from the agave cactus. It's a clear, light brown liquid, similar in appearance to maple syrup, though slightly thicker. It has a subtle, pleasant flavor and is very sweet, about twice as sweet as cane sugar. Because of its liquid form, it dissolves instantly, making it a great choice for sweetening beverages and dressings. Unlike honey, agave nectar is considered a vegan food.

This salad shines with a light and flavorful salt-free vinaigrette. For added protein, toss in a handful of sunflower seeds or chopped walnuts, or expand the salad into a one-dish meal by adding thinly sliced red onion, fresh green beans, or cooked barley. Adapted from *Eat, Drink & Be Vegan*.

1. Place unpeeled potatoes into a pot and add enough water to cover by a couple of inches. Bring to a boil over high heat. Once boiling, reduce heat to medium-high and simmer until tender, about 15 minutes.

2. Remove pot from heat and drain. Cut the potatoes into bite-sized chunks.

3. Place the potatoes back into the pot and add the spinach.

4. In a small bowl, whisk together the remaining ingredients, then pour over salad. Toss well to coat and combine.

5. Serve immediately or cover and refrigerate until ready to serve.

**Per Serving (1 cup)**

| | |
|---|---|
| Calories: 242 | Fiber: 4 grams |
| Fat: 9 grams | Carbohydrates: 37 grams |
| Protein: 4 grams | Sugar: 4 grams |
| Sodium: 20 milligrams | |

# Garlic Potato Salad

**Prep Time:** 10 minutes
**Cook Time:** 20 minutes
**Total Time:** 30 minutes
**Serves 6**

## INGREDIENTS

6 medium potatoes

3 cloves garlic, minced

1 cup sliced scallions

¼ cup olive oil

2 tablespoons unflavored rice vinegar

2 teaspoons chopped fresh rosemary

Freshly ground black pepper, to taste

This toothsome concoction of potatoes, scallions, and garlic is hefty enough to satisfy your hunger, yet light enough to not weigh you down. Use whichever type of potatoes you have on hand or like best. If you have the time, make this recipe ahead; the flavors improve the longer it sits. Either way, it's delicious. Adapted from *Simply in Season*.

1. Put the potatoes into a pot and add enough water to cover by 1 inch. Place over high heat and bring to a boil. Boil until fork tender but still solid; depending upon size, roughly 20 minutes.

2. Once cooked, remove from heat and place under cold running water. Drain and set potatoes aside to cool. Once cool enough to handle, cut into bite-sized cubes.

3. Place cubed potatoes, garlic, and scallions into a mixing bowl and toss to combine.

4. Measure the olive oil, vinegar, and rosemary into a small mixing bowl. Add freshly ground black pepper and whisk well to combine.

5. Pour the dressing over the salad and stir gently to coat. Serve immediately, or cover and refrigerate until serving.

**Per Serving (1 cup)**

Calories: 204

Fat: 9 grams

Protein: 2 grams

Sodium: 6 milligrams

Fiber: 2 grams

Carbohydrates: 28 grams

Sugar: 1 gram

# Veggie Pasta Salad with Zesty Italian Dressing

**Prep Time:** 15 minutes
**Cook Time:** 10 minutes
**Total Time:** 25 minutes
**Serves 12**

## INGREDIENTS

1 pound dry rotini (or similar pasta)

1 medium red onion, diced

2 cups grape tomatoes, halved

1 (15-ounce) can no-salt-added chickpeas, drained

⅓ cup low-sodium olives, sliced

1 medium cucumber, peeled, seeded, and diced

1 medium red bell pepper, diced

3 cups chopped fresh broccoli

1 small/medium yellow squash, diced

1 small/medium zucchini, diced

### DRESSING

4 tablespoons olive oil

4 tablespoons canola oil

4 tablespoons white vinegar

4 tablespoons apple cider vinegar

4 tablespoons water

1 teaspoon onion powder

1 teaspoon garlic powder

1½ teaspoons sugar

1½ teaspoons dried oregano

1 teaspoon dried parsley

1 teaspoon all-purpose salt-free seasoning

¼ teaspoon dried basil

¼ teaspoon freshly ground black pepper

⅛ teaspoon dried thyme

Perfect for potlucks, BBQs, and picnics, this pasta salad will be the hit of the party. This recipe makes enough to serve 12, so if you're feeding a smaller group, just halve the ingredients. The tangy dressing is also great on green salads or as a marinade for lean meat. If you can't find low-sodium olives at your local supermarket, buy them online.

1. Cook the pasta according to directions, omitting salt. Drain and set aside.

2. Prepare all of the veggies and place in an extra-large mixing bowl. Add pasta. Set aside.

3. Measure the dressing ingredients into a small mixing bowl and whisk well to combine.

4. Pour the dressing over the salad and toss well to coat. Serve immediately or cover and refrigerate until serving.

**Per Serving (1 cup)**

| | |
|---|---|
| Calories: 316 | Fiber: 5 grams |
| Fat: 10 grams | Carbohydrates: 45 grams |
| Protein: 9 grams | Sugar: 6 grams |
| Sodium: 18 milligrams | |

# Edamame Salad with Corn and Cranberries

**Prep Time:** 5 minutes
**Cook Time:** 0 minutes
**Total Time:** 5 minutes
**Serves 4**

## INGREDIENTS

1¼ cups shelled edamame

¾ cup fresh cooked or frozen (and thawed) corn kernels

1 small red or orange bell pepper, diced

¼ cup dried cranberries

1 shallot, finely diced

2 tablespoons red wine vinegar

1 tablespoon olive oil

1 teaspoon agave nectar

1 teaspoon no-salt-added prepared mustard

Freshly ground black pepper, to taste

A delightfully chewy, crisp, and colorful way to brighten plates and palates year round. This super-quick, low-sodium salad makes a great side, especially when served with sandwiches. If you can't find fresh corn on the cob or if it's out of season, just substitute an equal amount of thawed frozen corn. Either way, it tastes great!

1. Place the edamame, corn, bell pepper, cranberries, and shallot in a mixing bowl and stir to combine.

2. Measure the vinegar, olive oil, agave nectar, and mustard into a small mixing bowl and whisk well.

3. Pour the dressing over the salad and toss to coat. Season with freshly ground black pepper, to taste.

4. Serve immediately or cover and refrigerate until ready to serve.

**Per Serving (¾ cup)**
Calories: 149
Fat: 5 grams
Protein: 5 grams
Sodium: 5 milligrams

Fiber: 3 grams
Carbohydrates: 22 grams
Sugar: 10 grams

# The Best 3-Bean Salad *Ever!*

**Prep Time:** 5 minutes
**Cook Time:** 0 minutes
**Total Time:** 5 minutes
Serves 8

## INGREDIENTS

1 (15-ounce) can no-salt-added black beans

1 (15-ounce) can no-salt-added garbanzo beans

1 (15-ounce) can no-salt-added kidney beans

1 small onion, finely chopped

3 stalks celery, diced

⅓ cup canola oil

⅓ cup apple cider vinegar

⅓ cup agave nectar

Freshly ground black pepper, to taste

**To Bean or Not to Bean? That Shouldn't Be the Question!**

If you're having a hard time finding low-sodium canned beans at your local supermarket, don't let it discourage you from eating them altogether. Standard commercial beans are higher in sodium, but you can remove a lot of this excess by simply draining and rinsing them repeatedly in cold water.

I've always loved 3-bean salad. The sweet and sour tang of the dressing, the appealing interplay of texture and color. Unfortunately, most commercial versions are high in sodium and suffer from what I call "pickled syndrome"—flaccid ingredients bathed in a dressing that's sweeter than aspartame. I prefer 3-bean salad to soothe the palate, rather than attack it. This version is deliciously healthy, protein-packed, and ready in just 5 minutes!

1. Drain and rinse the beans, then place in a mixing bowl. Add the onion and celery. Stir to combine.

2. In a small mixing bowl, whisk together the oil, vinegar, and agave nectar. Pour over the salad and toss to coat. Season with freshly ground black pepper, to taste.

3. Serve immediately or cover and refrigerate until serving.

**Per Serving (1 cup)**

Calories: 313

Fat: 10 grams

Protein: 14 grams

Sodium: 19 milligrams

Fiber: 13 grams

Carbohydrates: 41 grams

Sugar: 4 grams

# Creamy Low-Sodium Coleslaw

**Prep Time:** 5 minutes
**Cook Time:** 0 minutes
**Total Time:** 5 minutes
**Serves 6**

## INGREDIENTS

½ medium-head green cabbage, shredded

1 medium carrot, shredded

1 small onion, grated

⅓ cup Salt-Free Mayonnaise (see recipe in this chapter)

3 tablespoons sugar

3 tablespoons apple cider vinegar

½ teaspoon dry ground mustard

½ teaspoon freshly ground black pepper

Your favorite picnic fare, low-sodium style! Cabbage, carrots, and grated onion caressed in a light and creamy dressing. If you don't have time to make your own Salt-Free Mayonnaise, try using nonfat sour cream instead. Before adding to the dish, measure the sour cream into a small bowl and beat in a teaspoon or two of prepared salt-free mustard. To further enhance the flavor, add a minced garlic clove, freshly squeezed lemon juice, and salt-free seasoning.

1. Combine all the ingredients in a large mixing bowl and stir well.

2. Cover and refrigerate until ready to serve.

**Per Serving (½ cup)**
Calories: 133
Fat: 8 grams
Protein: 2 grams
Sodium: 32 milligrams

Fiber: 3 grams
Carbohydrates: 13 grams
Sugar: 10 grams

# Salt-Free Mayonnaise

Prep Time: 5 minutes
Cook Time: 0 minutes
Total Time: 5 minutes
Yields 1 cup

## INGREDIENTS

¼ cup liquid egg substitute (e.g., Egg Beaters)

2½ tablespoons distilled white vinegar

½ teaspoon white pepper

⅛ teaspoon garlic powder

⅛ teaspoon dry ground mustard

Pinch ground cayenne pepper

⅔ cup canola oil

### Liquid Egg Substitutes

Sold in cartons alongside eggs, liquid egg substitutes such as Egg Beaters are a great way of enjoying the flavor of whole eggs without the fat and cholesterol. In most recipes, you can substitute ¼ cup of liquid egg substitute for each egg without a discernable difference in taste or texture. Liquid egg substitutes can be frozen as well, making them both healthy and convenient.

This light and creamy mayonnaise uses liquid egg substitute, eliminating both cholesterol and the risk of salmonella. Make this recipe ahead when you have time; homemade salt-free mayonnaise keeps well for a week if stored in a clean, airtight jar in the refrigerator. Adjust seasonings to suit your own taste. Adapted from *Southern Living* magazine.

1. Place all of the ingredients except the oil into a food processor and pulse until smooth. Scrape down sides.

2. With food processor running, add the oil in a slow and steady stream until mixture thickens.

3. Store mayonnaise in a clean, lidded jar and refrigerate when not in use.

**Per Serving (1 tablespoon)**
Calories: 84
Fat: 9 grams
Protein: 0 grams
Sodium: 7 milligrams

Fiber: 0 grams
Carbohydrates: 0 grams
Sugar: 0 grams

# Southwestern Beet Slaw

**Prep Time:** 15 minutes
**Cook Time:** 0 minutes
**Total Time:** 15 minutes
**Serves 6**

This simple salad will make a beet lover out of you!
Shredded beets are combined with carrots, scallions,
garlic, cilantro, and lime vinaigrette. The resulting
slaw is subtly sweet, spicy, and spectacular. If you do
not wish to have dyed hands for a day, wear a pair of
cheap, disposable gloves while making this recipe.

## INGREDIENTS

3 small/medium beets

3 scallions, sliced

2 medium carrots, shredded

¼ cup chopped fresh cilantro

2 cloves garlic, minced

Juice of 2 fresh limes

1 teaspoon olive oil

½ teaspoon salt-free chili seasoning

¼ teaspoon freshly ground black pepper

1. Trim and peel the beets, then shred. Place into a
   mixing bowl.

2. Add the scallions, carrots, cilantro, and garlic and
   stir well to combine.

3. In a small bowl, combine the lime juice, olive oil,
   chili seasoning, and black pepper and whisk well.
   Pour dressing over salad and toss well to coat.

4. Serve immediately or cover and refrigerate until
   ready to serve.

**Per Serving (½ cup)**

Calories: 38

Fat: 1 gram

Protein: 1 gram

Sodium: 46 milligrams

Fiber: 2 grams

Carbohydrates: 7 grams

Sugar: 4 grams

# Simple Autumn Salad

**Prep Time:** 10 minutes
**Cook Time:** 0 minutes
**Total Time:** 10 minutes
**Serves 4**

## INGREDIENTS

1 large head red leaf lettuce

1 pear, thinly sliced

½ small red onion, thinly sliced

½ cup dried black mission figs, chopped

⅓ cup chopped walnuts

2 tablespoons red or white balsamic vinegar

2 tablespoons olive oil

1 clove garlic, minced

¼ teaspoon freshly ground black pepper

A tasty combination of red leaf lettuce, red onion, pear, and walnuts in a light and tangy vinaigrette. This salad can be enjoyed any time of the year, simply by swapping out ingredients. Try nectarines or peaches in summer, apples in the fall, and strawberries in the spring. Whichever way you make it, it's salt-free, healthy, and delicious.

1. Wash the lettuce, pat dry, then tear into bite-sized pieces. Place in a bowl with the sliced pear, onion, figs, and walnuts. Set aside.

2. In a small bowl, add the vinegar, oil, garlic, and black pepper and whisk well to combine. Pour the dressing over the salad and toss to coat. Serve immediately.

**Per Serving (1½ cups)**

| | |
|---|---|
| Calories: 224 | Fiber: 5 grams |
| Fat: 14 grams | Carbohydrates: 25 grams |
| Protein: 3 grams | Sugar: 15 grams |
| Sodium: 29 milligrams | |

# Summer Corn Salad with Peppers and Avocado

**Prep Time:** 10 minutes
**Cook Time:** 0 minutes
**Total Time:** 10 minutes
**Serves 6**

## INGREDIENTS

2½ cups corn kernels (3 cooked fresh cobs, or frozen and thawed)

1 medium red bell pepper

1 ripe avocado

1 jalapeño pepper, minced

1 scallion, thinly sliced

1 clove garlic, minced

Juice of 1 fresh lime

2 tablespoons olive oil

Freshly ground black pepper, to taste

### Lend Me Your Ear!

Corn is high in vitamin C, is a great source of both protein and fiber, and contains antioxidants associated with reduced risk of cardiovascular disease and hypertension. It can be eaten hot or cold, on the cob or in single kernels, and even popped. Corn also grows easily in the home garden. Its sweet taste and vibrant color adds flavor, interest, and nutrition to any meal.

The next time you make corn on the cob, set a few ears aside for this fabulous summer salad. Or when time is tight and the weather is cold, simply substitute thawed frozen corn. The simple ingredients blend together so perfectly. And the lime juice—oh my! There is something about lime juice that makes even basic things taste festive.

1. If using fresh cooked corn, cut the kernels from the cob carefully using a very sharp knife. Place in a mixing bowl.

2. Core and dice the red pepper, then peel and dice the avocado. Add to the bowl, along with the jalapeño, sliced scallion (white and green parts), and minced garlic.

3. In a small bowl, whisk together the lime juice and olive oil. Drizzle over the salad and toss to coat. Season to taste with freshly ground black pepper.

4. Serve immediately or cover and refrigerate until ready to serve.

**Per Serving (1 cup)**
Calories: 135
Fat: 9 grams
Protein: 2 grams
Sodium: 5 milligrams
Fiber: 3 grams
Carbohydrates: 13 grams
Sugar: 2 grams

# Curried Tofu Salad

**Prep Time:** 10 minutes
**Cook Time:** 5 minutes
**Total Time:** 15 minutes
Serves 6

## INGREDIENTS

1 pound extra-firm tofu, drained and cubed

3 medium stalks celery, diced

1 small green apple, diced

1 small red apple, diced

¾ cup golden raisins

¼ cup chopped walnuts

3 tablespoons apple cider vinegar

2 tablespoons canola oil

1 teaspoon salt-free curry powder

⅛ teaspoon ground cumin

¼ teaspoon freshly ground black pepper

A curried twist on the classic Waldorf salad, this vegan version adds the heft and protein of tofu but swaps mayonnaise for a lighter vinaigrette. If you're someone who avoids tofu, just substitute an equal amount of cooked chicken. Adapted from *Eating Well When You Just Can't Eat the Way You Used To.*

1. Place the tofu into the steamer basket of a pot or appliance and steam for 5 minutes. Remove and set aside to cool.

2. Place the celery, apples, raisins, and walnuts into a mixing bowl and add the tofu when it has cooled to touch.

3. Measure the remaining ingredients into a small bowl and whisk well to combine. Drizzle the dressing over the salad and toss gently to coat.

4. Serve immediately or cover and refrigerate until ready to serve.

**Per Serving (1 cup)**

| | |
|---|---|
| Calories: 226 | Fiber: 3 grams |
| Fat: 12 grams | Carbohydrates: 23 grams |
| Protein: 9 grams | Sugar: 15 grams |
| Sodium: 22 milligrams | |

# Tart Apple Salad with Honey Yogurt Dressing

**Prep Time:** 10 minutes
**Cook Time:** 0 minutes
**Total Time:** 10 minutes
Serves 6

## INGREDIENTS

2 tart green apples, diced

1 small bulb fennel, including stalk and fronds, chopped

1½ cups seedless red grapes, halved

2 tablespoons freshly squeezed lemon juice

¼ cup low-fat vanilla yogurt

1 teaspoon honey

Crunchy and sweet with a light, refreshing finish. The fennel really makes this salad and can be used in its entirety—bulb, stalks, and fronds. Leave the peel on the apples for added nutrients and fiber. If you can't find fennel, or simply don't care for its licorice taste, substitute an equal amount of chopped celery.

1. Measure all the ingredients into a mixing bowl and stir well to combine.

2. Serve immediately or cover and refrigerate until ready to serve.

**Per Serving (1 cup)**

Calories: 70
Fat: <1 gram
Protein: 1 gram
Sodium: 26 milligrams

Fiber: 3 grams
Carbohydrates: 16 grams
Sugar: 11 grams

### Fennel Facts

Fennel is a vegetable with the pronounced flavor and aroma of anise (black licorice). Every part of the plant is edible and can be eaten either raw or cooked. Fennel has a firm white bulb from which green celery-like stalks grow, topped with soft, dill-like fronds. When it blossoms, its flowers produce small, edible, anise-flavored seeds. Fennel is high in fiber and protein, is said to alleviate stomach upset and gas, and contains antioxidants linked to preventing heart disease and cancer.

# Whole-Wheat Couscous Salad with Citrus and Cilantro

**Prep Time:** 5 minutes
**Cook Time:** 7 minutes
**Total Time:** 12 minutes
**Serves 6**

## INGREDIENTS

1½ cups water

1 cup whole-wheat couscous

1 medium cucumber

1 pint grape or cherry tomatoes, halved

1 jalapeño pepper, minced

2 shallots, minced

2 scallions, sliced

2 cloves garlic, minced

2 tablespoons freshly squeezed lemon juice

2 tablespoons freshly squeezed lime juice

1 teaspoon olive oil

¼ cup chopped fresh cilantro

Freshly ground black pepper, to taste

This whole-grain salad strikes the perfect balance between light and filling. Its refreshing taste can be enjoyed year round, but is best in summer with fresh-picked garden produce. Couscous is a tiny grain-like pasta made from semolina (wheat) flour. It cooks in minutes and makes an easy and convenient alternative to rice and other grains. Couscous comes in white and whole-wheat varieties; the whole-wheat version has the added benefits of whole grain, thus making it a healthier choice. If you can't find couscous, or have an allergy to gluten, feel free to substitute cooked quinoa instead.

1. Measure water into a saucepan and bring to a boil over high heat. Once boiling, stir in the couscous, reduce heat to medium-low, cover, and simmer for 2 minutes.

2. Remove pot from heat, remove lid, and fluff couscous with a fork. Set aside to cool for 5 minutes.

3. Peel the cucumber and slice in half lengthwise. Use a spoon to gently scrape out the seeds, then dice and place into a mixing bowl.

4. Add the remaining ingredients to the bowl along with the cooked couscous and toss well to coat.

5. Season to taste with freshly ground black pepper. Serve immediately or cover and refrigerate until ready to serve.

**Per Serving (1 cup)**
Calories: 126
Fat: 2 grams
Protein: 4 grams
Sodium: 5 milligrams

Fiber: 2 grams
Carbohydrates: 24 grams
Sugar: 3 grams

# Tomato, Cucumber, and Basil Salad

**Prep Time:** 10 minutes
**Cook Time:** 0 minutes
**Total Time:** 10 minutes
**Serves 4**

## INGREDIENTS

2 small/medium cucumbers

4 ripe medium tomatoes, quartered

1 small onion, thinly sliced

¼ cup chopped fresh basil

3 tablespoons red wine vinegar

1 tablespoon olive oil

1 clove garlic, minced

¼ teaspoon freshly ground black pepper

Savor the taste of summer with ripe, garden-fresh produce covered in a tangy vinaigrette. If you have time, make this salad ahead, cover, and refrigerate until serving. The longer the flavors are allowed to steep, the better it tastes. Add a can of drained and rinsed chickpeas to the mix for a heartier one-dish meal.

1. Peel the cucumbers, slice in half lengthwise, then use a spoon to gently scrape out the seeds.

2. Slice the cucumber halves and place in a bowl. Add the tomatoes, onion, and basil.

3. Place the remaining ingredients into a small bowl and whisk well to combine.

4. Pour the dressing over the salad and toss to coat. Serve immediately or cover and refrigerate until ready to serve.

**Per Serving (1 cup)**
Calories: 66
Fat: 4 grams
Protein: 1 gram
Sodium: 9 milligrams

Fiber: 2 grams
Carbohydrates: 7 grams
Sugar: 4 grams

# Tropical Chicken Salad

Prep Time: 5 minutes
Cook Time: 20 minutes
Total Time: 25 minutes
Serves 6

## INGREDIENTS

1 pound boneless, skinless chicken breast

2 tablespoons apple cider vinegar

Juice of 1 freshly squeezed lime

2 tablespoons olive oil

¼ cup chopped fresh cilantro

½ teaspoon ground white pepper

1 ripe mango, diced

1 small red onion, diced

1 small bell pepper, diced

1 jalapeño pepper, minced

2 cloves garlic, minced

1 cup cooked no-salt-added black beans

Perfect for warm weather, this new take on the classic picnic fare is colorfully festive and has a fresh, spicy kick. This recipe replaces artery-clogging mayonnaise with a light, delicious vinaigrette, which is fabulous on its own, over a bed of greens, or as a filling for wrap sandwiches. Serve with sliced avocado if desired.

1. Place chicken breast into a pot and add enough water to cover. Bring to a boil over high heat. Once boiling, reduce heat slightly, and continue boiling about 20 minutes, until fully cooked. Remove from heat, drain, and set aside to cool.

2. While the chicken is cooling, place the vinegar, lime juice, olive oil, cilantro, and white pepper into a small bowl and whisk well to combine.

3. Once the chicken is cool to touch, cut into bite-sized pieces. Place into a mixing bowl and add the mango, onion, peppers, garlic, and beans. Pour the dressing over the chicken salad and stir well to coat.

4. Serve immediately or cover and refrigerate until serving.

**Per Serving (1 cup)**
Calories: 194
Fat: 6 grams
Protein: 20 grams
Sodium: 52 milligrams
Fiber: 3 grams
Carbohydrates: 15 grams
Sugar: 6 grams

# Lemon Vinaigrette

**Prep Time:** 2 minutes
**Cook Time:** 0 minutes
**Total Time:** 2 minutes
**Yields 3 ounces**

## INGREDIENTS

¼ cup freshly squeezed lemon juice

1 tablespoon olive oil

1 tablespoon minced fresh shallot

1 tablespoon honey

Freshly ground black pepper, to taste

Get ready to lick your plate! This irresistibly zesty dressing adds sparkle to salads and makes a great marinade for veggies, meat, and tofu. Instead of lemon juice, try substituting lime or key lime, grapefruit, orange, or tangerine juice. Add a tablespoon of chopped fresh mint. Trade minced ginger or sliced scallion for the shallot. Or use agave nectar instead of the honey.

1. Place all the ingredients into a small bowl and whisk well to combine.

2. Use immediately or cover and refrigerate until ready to serve.

**Per Serving (1 ounce)**

| | |
|---|---|
| Calories: 69 | Fiber: 0 grams |
| Fat: 4 grams | Carbohydrates: 8 grams |
| Protein: 0 grams | Sugar: 6 grams |
| Sodium: 0 grams | |

# Sesame Ginger Vinaigrette

**Prep Time:** 2 minutes
**Cook Time:** ½ minute
**Total Time:** 2½ minutes
**Yields ⅔ cup**

## INGREDIENTS

¼ cup unflavored rice wine vinegar

1 tablespoon sesame oil

1 tablespoon minced fresh ginger

2 cloves garlic, minced

1 teaspoon sugar

¼ teaspoon ground white pepper

Modeled after the ginger dressing served at my favorite Japanese restaurant, this low-sodium vinaigrette will have you craving salads like never before. Use it to dress a salad of mixed greens, slivered carrot and radish, ripe tomato, pea pods, and thinly sliced cucumber. Sprinkle with toasted almonds, sesame seeds, or dried seaweed.

1. Place all of the ingredients into a small microwave-safe bowl and whisk well to combine.

2. Microwave for 30 seconds on high, then remove and whisk well again.

3. Pour over salad and toss well to coat. Serve immediately.

**Per Serving (2 tablespoons)**

Calories: 58
Fat: 5 grams
Protein: 0 grams
Sodium: 0 milligrams

Fiber: 0 grams
Carbohydrates: 2 grams
Sugar: 1 gram

# Tomato Garlic Dressing

**Prep Time:** 2 minutes
**Cook Time:** 0 minutes
**Total Time:** 2 minutes
**Yields** ⅔ cup

## INGREDIENTS

2 tablespoons red wine vinegar

2 tablespoons lemon juice

1 tablespoon salt-free tomato paste

1½ teaspoons olive oil

2 cloves garlic

1 teaspoon agave nectar

¼ teaspoon freshly ground black pepper

### Homemade Dressing

Store-bought salad dressings offer convenience, but at what cost? Most are filled with fat, excess sodium, sugar, and unrecognizable ingredients. Instead of buying commercial dressings, spend your money on new and interesting vinegars, oils, and fruit juices. Then for a world of flavor in just minutes, add garlic, scallions, or shallot, fresh or dried herbs, ground or prepared mustard, and other spices.

If you're someone who puts ketchup on everything, here's the low-fat dressing of your dreams! With its vibrant color and tangy taste, it's great drizzled over salad or served with grilled vegetables, meats, and sandwiches. Try it as a salt-free marinade to perk up your favorite protein.

1. Place all of the ingredients into a food processor and pulse until smooth.

2. Serve immediately or store in an airtight container until ready to serve.

**Per Serving (2 tablespoons)**

Calories: 60

Fat: 2 grams

Protein: 0 grams

Sodium: 7 milligrams

Fiber: 0 grams

Carbohydrates: 9 grams

Sugar: 7 grams

# Apple Honey Mustard Vinaigrette

**Prep Time:** 2 minutes
**Cook Time:** 0 minutes
**Total Time:** 2 minutes
**Yields ½ cup**

## INGREDIENTS

¼ cup apple cider vinegar

2 tablespoons honey

1 tablespoon olive oil

1 teaspoon dry ground mustard

¼ teaspoon freshly ground black pepper

Toss this sweet, tangy dressing with salad greens or use it to sauté spinach, Swiss chard, or kale. For a twist on this dressing, add some minced garlic or a squeeze of lemon juice. You really can't go wrong with home-made dressing. Let your imagination guide you.

1. Place all the ingredients into a small bowl and whisk well to combine.

2. Serve immediately or cover and refrigerate until ready to serve.

**Per Serving (2 tablespoons)**

| | |
|---|---|
| Calories: 65 | Fiber: 0 grams |
| Fat: 3 grams | Carbohydrates: 9 grams |
| Protein: 0 grams | Sugar: 8 grams |
| Sodium: 1 milligram | |

# CHAPTER 4

# Sandwiches and Soups

# Grilled Chicken Patties

**Prep Time:** 5 minutes
**Cook Time:** 12 minutes
**Total Time:** 17 minutes
**Serves 4**

## INGREDIENTS

1 pound lean ground chicken

1 teaspoon ground sweet paprika

½ teaspoon freshly ground black pepper

½ teaspoon ground cumin

½ teaspoon salt-free chili seasoning

¼ teaspoon dried red pepper flakes

### Keeping Grilled Burgers Juicy

Burgers have a tendency to round upward while cooking on the grill. To keep patties flat while cooking, make a small indentation in the center of each side using the back of a spoon or your thumb. The indented centers will rise to meet the rest of the burger, without the need for flattening the whole thing down with a spatula. Grilled burgers will remain juicy and delicious!

Lean ground chicken and Southwestern spices make one yummy burger. Best of all, they're so low in sodium that you can splurge: sandwich these patties between whole-grain buns! Serve with thick slices of ripe tomato, lettuce, and a slice of low-sodium Swiss cheese for a healthy take on the all-American meal.

1. Preheat grill.

2. Place ground chicken into a mixing bowl. Add the seasonings and mix thoroughly using your hands. Divide mixture into 4 equal portions. Roll each portion into a ball, then flatten to form patties.

3. Once grill is ready, place patties on surface. Grill for 5–6 minutes on the first side, then gently flip patties and grill for another 5–6 minutes on the second side. For well-done patties, a safe internal temperature is 170°F.

4. Remove from grill, place on buns if desired, and serve immediately.

**Per Serving (1 patty)**
Calories: 118
Fat: 2 grams
Protein: 20 grams
Sodium: 73 milligrams

Fiber: 0 grams
Carbohydrates: 1 gram
Sugar: 0 grams

# Ground Turkey Sloppy Joes

**Prep Time:** 5 minutes
**Cook Time:** 25 minutes
**Total Time:** 30 minutes
**Serves 4**

## INGREDIENTS

1 pound lean ground turkey

1 medium onion, diced

3 cloves garlic, minced

1 medium red bell pepper, diced

1 medium tomato, diced

1 (8-ounce) can no-salt-added tomato sauce

1 (6-ounce) can salt-free tomato paste

¼ cup apple cider vinegar

2 tablespoons brown sugar

1 teaspoon dried oregano

½ teaspoon ground cumin

Freshly ground black pepper, to taste

4 Soft and Crusty No-Rise Sandwich Rolls (see recipe in this chapter)

Tangy, sweet, and slightly sour, these sloppy joes are every bit as good as the salty ones you used to enjoy. Lean ground chicken or beef can be substituted for the turkey if desired. Although these are fabulous served as sandwiches, the filling also tastes great spooned over cooked rice and other grains, baked potatoes, or pasta.

1. Place the ground turkey, onion, and garlic in a sauté pan over medium heat. Cook, stirring, for 5 minutes.

2. Add remaining ingredients and stir to combine. Reduce heat to medium-low and simmer for 20 minutes, stirring occasionally. Remove from heat.

3. Divide mixture evenly between rolls. Serve immediately.

**Per Serving (1¼ cups filling and 1 roll)**

| | |
|---|---|
| Calories: 407 | Fiber: 6 grams |
| Fat: 9 grams | Carbohydrates: 52 grams |
| Protein: 30 grams | Sugar: 18 grams |
| Sodium: 142 milligrams | |

# Tofu Sloppy Joes

**Prep Time:** 10 minutes
**Cook Time:** 13 minutes
**Total Time:** 23 minutes
**Serves 4**

## INGREDIENTS

1 pound extra-firm tofu

2 teaspoons canola oil

1 medium onion, diced

1 medium bell pepper, diced

1 medium stalk celery, diced

2 (8-ounce) cans no-salt-added tomato sauce

1½ tablespoons apple cider vinegar

1 tablespoon salt-free prepared mustard

¾ teaspoon low-sodium Worcestershire sauce

1 teaspoon sugar

Freshly ground black pepper, to taste

4 Soft and Crusty No-Rise Sandwich Rolls (see recipe in this chapter)

*If you're skeptical of tofu, give this recipe a try. With sautéed veggies, tomato sauce, and a vinegar tang, it's transformed into something so delicious, you'll be asking for seconds. This filling tastes great on sandwich buns, spooned over cooked rice or quinoa, or stuffed into baked potatoes. If you have time, freeze the tofu the night before cooking, then thaw and drain. Freezing changes the texture of the tofu, making it more dense and meat-like. Adapted from Prevention's The Healthy Cook.*

1. Drain tofu and press firmly between 2 plates to release any additional liquid. Pat dry with paper towels, then crumble the tofu coarsely with a fork or your fingers.

2. Heat the oil in a sauté pan over medium heat. Add the tofu, onions, bell pepper, and celery and sauté for 8 minutes.

3. Stir in the tomato sauce, vinegar, mustard, Worcestershire sauce, and sugar. Cook, stirring frequently, for 5 minutes.

4. Remove from heat and season to taste with freshly ground black pepper. Divide the mixture evenly between the buns. Serve immediately.

**Per Serving (1¼ cups filling and 1 roll)**

| | |
|---|---|
| Calories: 348 | Fiber: 6 grams |
| Fat: 1 gram | Carbohydrates: 45 grams |
| Protein: 18 grams | Sugar: 10 grams |
| Sodium: 46 milligrams | |

# Salmon Cakes

Prep Time: 10 minutes
Cook Time: 15 minutes
Total Time: 25 minutes
Serves 6

## INGREDIENTS

1 (15-ounce) can no-salt-added boneless salmon

4 tablespoons Salt-Free Mayonnaise (see Chapter 3: Salads and Dressings)

½ cup salt-free bread crumbs

1 small onion, chopped finely

1 small bell pepper, chopped finely

1 egg white

1 teaspoon dried herbes de Provence

½ teaspoon ground sweet paprika

¼ teaspoon dry ground mustard

⅛ teaspoon celery seed

Freshly ground black pepper, to taste

### Mayonnaise Substitute

Instead of adding Salt-Free Mayonnaise to a recipe like this one, try substituting an equal amount of plain nonfat Greek yogurt. Its thick and creamy consistency works well in many types of salads and sandwiches, from tuna and salmon to chicken and egg. To thin the yogurt, add a little lemon juice or low-sodium broth. For added flavor, add minced garlic and some chopped fresh herbs.

Thanks to Healthy Heart Market, Trader Joe's, Whole Foods Market, and others, you can buy canned salt-free salmon without difficulty or tremendous expense. If you can't find it locally, no-salt-added canned tuna can be substituted instead. Delicately crisp outside and flavorfully moist inside, these salmon cakes are a real treat sandwiched in rolls or enjoyed plain.

1. Preheat oven to 400°F. Spray a baking sheet lightly with oil and set aside.

2. Drain salmon well and place into a mixing bowl. Add remaining ingredients and mix well using a spoon or your hands. Divide mixture into 6 equal portions and shape into patties.

3. Arrange patties on the prepared baking sheet then place it on middle rack in oven and bake for 10 minutes. Remove from oven, gently flip patties, and return to oven to bake 5 minutes more.

4. Remove from oven and serve immediately.

**Per Serving (1 patty)**

| | |
|---|---|
| Calories: 202 | Fiber: 1 gram |
| Fat: 11 grams | Carbohydrates: 8 grams |
| Protein: 16 grams | Sugar: 1 gram |
| Sodium: 68 milligrams | |

# Black Bean Burgers

Prep Time: 10 minutes
Cook Time: 15 minutes
Total Time: 25 minutes
Serves 4

## INGREDIENTS

2 (15-ounce) cans no-salt-added black beans

½ cup salt-free bread crumbs

1 shallot, minced

3 cloves garlic, minced

1 medium red bell pepper, chopped

¼ cup chopped fresh cilantro

1 tablespoon freshly squeezed lime juice

2 teaspoons salt-free chili seasoning

Freshly ground black pepper, to taste

This hearty homemade veggie burger is packed with Southwestern flavor. Low-fat, low-sodium, and cholesterol-free, these patties are high in fiber and take less than 30 minutes to prepare. They taste great on buns and garnished with homemade guacamole and salsa. Pair this zesty dish with fresh corn and cooked brown rice tossed with lime juice and chopped cilantro.

1. Preheat oven to 425°F. Spray a baking sheet lightly with oil and set aside.

2. Drain and rinse the beans, then place in a food processor and purée until smooth.

3. Transfer the beans to a mixing bowl, add remaining ingredients, then mix together using your hands. Form into 4 large patties.

4. Arrange patties on prepared baking sheet then place it on middle rack in oven and bake for 10 minutes. Remove from oven, gently flip patties, and return to oven. Bake for another 5 minutes.

5. Remove from oven and serve immediately.

**Per Serving (1 patty)**

| | |
|---|---|
| Calories: 348 | Fiber: 13 grams |
| Fat: 1 gram | Carbohydrates: 69 grams |
| Protein: 19 grams | Sugar: 3 grams |
| Sodium: 11 milligrams | |

# Spinach Burgers

**Prep Time:** 10 minutes
**Cook Time:** 20 minutes
**Total Time:** 30 minutes
**Serves 4**

## INGREDIENTS

1 teaspoon olive oil

1 medium red onion, diced

4 cloves garlic, minced

1 medium red bell pepper, diced

6 cups fresh baby spinach, chopped

1½ teaspoons dried Italian seasoning

½ teaspoon freshly ground black pepper

1 egg white

¼ cup shredded Swiss cheese

½ cup salt-free bread crumbs

A different way to enjoy your spinach, these burgers are thick, hearty, and completely vegetarian. The shredded Swiss cheese enhances the flavor of the burgers while keeping the sodium low. For delicious gluten-free burgers, substitute cooked quinoa for the salt-free bread crumbs. Serve with sautéed mushrooms, with or without buns.

1. Preheat oven to 425°F. Spray a baking sheet lightly with oil and set aside.

2. Heat olive oil in a sauté pan over medium heat. Add the onion, garlic, and bell pepper and sauté for 3 minutes.

3. Add the spinach and sauté until wilted, about 2 minutes more. Remove pan from heat.

4. Add the Italian seasoning and black pepper. Stir well, scraping up the brown bits from the bottom of the pan. Allow to cool for 5 minutes.

5. Add egg white, Swiss cheese, and bread crumbs to pan and stir well to combine. Form mixture into 4 patties.

6. Arrange patties on prepared baking sheet, then place it on middle rack in oven and bake for 10 minutes. Flip patties and bake an additional 5 minutes.

7. Remove from oven and serve immediately.

**Per Serving (1 patty)**
Calories: 111
Fat: 3 grams
Protein: 6 grams
Sodium: 66 milligrams

Fiber: 2 grams
Carbohydrates: 15 grams
Sugar: 1 gram

# Beef and Bean Tacos

**Prep Time:** 10 minutes
**Cook Time:** 15 minutes
**Total Time:** 25 minutes
**Serves 6**

## INGREDIENTS

1 package (12 tacos) low-sodium taco shells

1 pound extra-lean ground beef

1 medium onion, diced finely

1 jalapeño pepper, minced

2 cloves garlic, minced

1 (15-ounce) can no-salt-added black beans

⅔ cup fresh or frozen (and thawed) corn kernels

1 tablespoon salt-free tomato ketchup

1 tablespoon salt-free tomato paste

1 teaspoon honey

¾ teaspoon liquid smoke

1½ teaspoons ground cumin

1 teaspoon ground sweet paprika

½ teaspoon ground coriander

½ teaspoon dry ground mustard

1 cup low-sodium tomato salsa

½ cup nonfat sour cream

¼ cup chopped fresh cilantro

### It's a Low-Sodium Fiesta at Trader Joe's!

Trader Joe's markets offer some of the best low-sodium fixings nationwide. Look for low-sodium taco shells, lightly salted or salt-free tortilla chips, salt-free salsa, and more at your nearest location. If you don't have a Trader Joe's close to home, check online purveyors such as *www.healthyheart market.com.*

These tacos are so tasty, you'll hardly believe they're low in sodium. Store any leftover filling in the fridge and it'll be as good or even better the next day. If you run out of taco shells, simply warm the filling and serve alongside salsa, sour cream, and unsalted tortilla chips for a delicious new take on nachos.

1. Heat the taco shells according to package directions.

2. Place the ground beef in a skillet or sauté pan over medium heat. Add the onion, jalapeño, and garlic and sauté for 5 minutes.

3. Drain the black beans and add to the pan, along with the corn, ketchup, tomato paste, honey, liquid smoke, and seasonings. Reduce heat to medium-low, and cook for 10 minutes, stirring frequently. Remove from heat.

4. Place heated taco shells on a clean surface and divide filling evenly between them. Top each with salsa, sour cream, and chopped cilantro.

5. Serve immediately.

**Per Serving (2 tacos)**
Calories: 388
Fat: 10 grams
Protein: 25 grams
Sodium: 182 milligrams
Fiber: 6 grams
Carbohydrates: 50 grams
Sugar: 8 grams

# Sweet Potato and Black Bean Tacos

**Prep Time:** 5 minutes
**Cook Time:** 25 minutes
**Total Time:** 30 minutes
**Serves 4**

## INGREDIENTS

1 package (12 tacos) low-sodium taco shells

3 small/medium sweet potatoes

1 tablespoon canola oil

1 medium onion, diced

¾ cup unsweetened apple juice, divided

1 (15-ounce) can no-salt-added black beans

1 teaspoon ground cumin

½ teaspoon ground cinnamon

½ teaspoon salt-free chili seasoning

Freshly ground black pepper, to taste

¼ cup low-sodium salsa

¼ cup nonfat sour cream

¼ cup chopped fresh cilantro

From stovetop to table in just 30 minutes, this recipe is an irresistible combination of sweet and savory flavors and textures. Each taco is dotted with luscious nonfat sour cream, spicy salsa, and the bite of cilantro. Make it a complete meal by serving them with cooked brown rice or quinoa tossed with lime juice. Adapted from *Simply in Season*.

1. Heat the taco shells according to package directions.

2. Peel the sweet potatoes and cut into ½-inch cubes.

3. Heat the oil in a sauté pan over medium heat. Add the diced sweet potato, onion, and ½ cup apple juice to the pan and stir to combine. Cover the pan and cook, stirring frequently, until sweet potatoes are tender, about 20 minutes.

4. Drain the black beans. Uncover the pan and add the beans, the remaining apple juice, and seasonings and stir to combine. Cook, stirring, for 5 minutes. Remove pan from heat.

5. Place the heated taco shells on a clean surface and divide filling evenly between them. Top each with salsa, sour cream, and chopped cilantro.

6. Serve immediately.

**Per Serving (3 tacos)**
Calories: 464
Fat: 13 grams
Protein: 14 grams
Sodium: 68 milligrams

Fiber: 13 grams
Carbohydrates: 75 grams
Sugar: 12 grams

# Refried Beans in 2 Minutes Flat

**Prep Time:** 2 minutes
**Cook Time:** 0 minutes
**Total Time:** 2 minutes
**Serves 3**

## INGREDIENTS

1 (15-ounce) can no-salt-added pinto, kidney, or black beans

1 teaspoon onion powder

½ teaspoon garlic powder

¼ teaspoon ground cumin

¼ teaspoon low-sodium soy sauce

Freshly ground black pepper, to taste

This fat-free, cholesterol-free, low-sodium, and incredibly tasty recipe comes together so fast, you can enjoy it any time the craving hits! Roll it up in tortillas with roasted veggies, or use as a spread for crackers and raw vegetables. Any type of canned beans will do: pinto, kidney, or black. If you can't find salt-free beans and don't have the time to cook your own, just use the standard canned kind, but be sure to drain and rinse well to eliminate as much sodium as possible. Adapted from *Mayim's Vegan Table*.

1. Drain and rinse the beans.

2. Place all of the ingredients into a food processor and pulse until smooth.

3. Serve immediately. Warm if desired, by placing in a microwave-safe bowl and heating for 1–2 minutes in the microwave, or spooning into a small saucepan and heating on low for 5 minutes on the stovetop.

**Per Serving (⅔ cup)**
Calories: 193
Fat: 1 gram
Protein: 12 grams
Sodium: 17 milligrams

Fiber: 12 grams
Carbohydrates: 35 grams
Sugar: 0 grams

# Barbecued Tempeh Sandwiches

**Prep Time:** 10 minutes
**Cook Time:** 20 minutes
**Total Time:** 30 minutes
**Serves 6**

## INGREDIENTS

2 teaspoons olive oil

1 (8-ounce) package organic tempeh, diced

1 large onion, diced

1 medium bell pepper, diced

3 cloves garlic, minced

1 (15-ounce) can no-salt-added diced tomatoes

2 (8-ounce) cans no-salt-added tomato sauce

1 tablespoon apple cider vinegar

1 tablespoon molasses

1½ teaspoons low-sodium Worcestershire sauce

1 teaspoon ground sweet paprika

½ teaspoon freshly ground black pepper

½ teaspoon ground cumin

¼ teaspoon ground cinnamon

¼ teaspoon liquid smoke

⅛ teaspoon ground cayenne pepper

¼ cup chopped fresh cilantro

6 Soft and Crusty No-Rise Sandwich Rolls (see recipe in this chapter)

These yummy sandwiches are a low-sodium take on vegan sloppy joes. While the recipe calls for serving the filling in buns, it's also delicious spooned over cooked brown rice, baked potatoes or sweet potatoes, pasta, egg-free noodles, couscous, or quinoa. Whatever you decide, this dish makes a quick and tasty meal, and is as filling as it is flavorful.

1. Heat olive oil in a sauté pan over medium heat. Add tempeh, onion, bell pepper, and garlic and sauté for 5 minutes.

2. Add remaining ingredients except for the cilantro. Reduce heat to medium-low, and cook for another 15 minutes, stirring frequently. Remove from heat.

3. Stir in cilantro and spoon tempeh mixture into buns. Serve immediately.

**Per Serving (1 cup filling and 1 roll)**

| | |
|---|---|
| Calories: 297 | Fiber: 5 grams |
| Fat: 8 grams | Carbohydrates: 45 grams |
| Protein: 14 grams | Sugar: 10 grams |
| Sodium: 44 milligrams | |

### What Is Tempeh?

Tempeh is a fermented soybean product sold in firm, rectangular cakes. It has a rugged texture and nutty flavor that melds well with many types of food. Cut it into cubes and add to pasta sauce, sauté along with vegetables, or marinate in your favorite sauce and bake. Tempeh is cholesterol-free and a good source of protein, calcium, and iron. Look for it in the grocery store produce section; it's typically stocked alongside the tofu.

# Meaty Portabella Burgers

Prep Time: 2 minutes
Cook Time: 13 minutes
Total Time: 15 minutes
Serves 4

## INGREDIENTS

4 large portabella mushroom caps

1 tablespoon olive oil

4 Soft and Crusty No-Rise Sandwich Rolls
(see recipe in this chapter)

Nothing satisfies hunger better than a burger, and this recipe proves you don't need meat to make the best burgers of your life. Portabella mushrooms are nature's veggie burgers. They're thick, patty-shaped, and even *brown!* When grilled, these large mushroom caps take on a great barbecue flavor, and their meaty heft becomes tender and indescribably juicy. Sandwiched in a bun with all your favorite toppings, you won't miss the meat.

1. Preheat grill to high.

2. Remove stems from mushrooms and discard. Brush mushroom caps with oil. Place gill side down on grill and cook for 8 minutes. Flip mushrooms over and grill another 5 minutes.

3. Remove mushrooms from grill and sandwich between rolls. Garnish with condiments of choice. Serve immediately.

**Per Serving (1 mushroom and 1 roll)**

| | |
|---|---|
| Calories: 201 | Fiber: 4 grams |
| Fat: 5 grams | Carbohydrates: 32 grams |
| Protein: 7 grams | Sugar: 3 grams |
| Sodium: 14 milligrams | |

# Soft and Crusty No-Rise Sandwich Rolls

**Prep Time:** 10 minutes
**Cook Time:** 20 minutes
**Total Time:** 30 minutes
**Yields 8 sandwich rolls or 12 dinner rolls**

## INGREDIENTS

1 tablespoon active dry yeast

2 teaspoons olive oil

1 tablespoon sugar

1 teaspoon all-purpose salt-free seasoning

1¼ cups warm water

1¼ cups unbleached all-purpose flour

1 cup white whole-wheat flour

1 large beaten egg, for brushing

### All-Purpose Salt-Free Seasoning

If there's a single seasoning you'll want to find for your low-sodium diet, it's this one! All-purpose salt-free seasoning is a unique blend of herbs, spices, dehydrated vegetables, citrus zest, and sometimes nutritional yeast. Its combination of flavors can replace salt both at the table and in recipes. My favorites are Benson's Table Tasty No Potassium Chloride Salt Substitute, Olde Thompson Organic No Salt Seasoning, and McCormick Perfect Pinch Salt Free Garlic & Herb Seasoning.

Low-sodium dieters despair no more! This quick and easy recipe yields fabulous sandwich rolls in just half an hour from start to finish! Brushing the bread with beaten egg before baking gives it a gloriously glossy, golden crust. The dough can be divided into 8 sandwich-sized rolls or 12 smaller dinner rolls. You can also bake the dough as a whole loaf—simply place in a small oiled pan and increase bake time to 30 minutes.

1. Preheat oven to 425°F. Spray a baking sheet lightly with oil and set aside.

2. Place the yeast, olive oil, sugar, and seasoning into a large mixing bowl and add the water. Gradually add in the flours, stirring well to combine.

3. Once dough comes together, turn out onto a lightly floured surface and knead, adding up to ¼ cup additional flour as necessary. Knead 5 minutes, until dough is smooth and elastic.

4. Shape loaf as desired or cut into 8 or 12 equal portions and roll into buns or rolls. Place on prepared baking sheet and brush lightly with beaten egg.

5. Place sheet on middle rack in oven and bake 15 minutes for 12 dinner rolls, or 20 minutes for 8 sandwich rolls.

6. Remove from oven and serve immediately, or transfer to a wire rack to cool.

**Per Serving (1 dinner roll)**

| | |
|---|---|
| Calories: 100 | Fiber: 1 gram |
| Fat: 1 gram | Carbohydrates: 18 grams |
| Protein: 3 grams | Sugar: 1 gram |
| Sodium: 7 milligrams | |

# Classic Chicken Noodle Soup

**Prep Time:** 10 minutes
**Cook Time:** 13 minutes
**Total Time:** 23 minutes
**Serves 4**

## INGREDIENTS

2 cups cooked, shredded chicken

2 medium carrots, sliced

1 medium stalk celery, sliced

1 small onion, diced

3 cloves garlic, minced

4 cups low-sodium chicken broth

2 teaspoons all-purpose salt-free seasoning

½ teaspoon ground sage

¼ teaspoon ground rosemary

Freshly ground black pepper, to taste

1½ cups yolkless egg noodles

The beauty of chicken noodle soup is in its simplicity, warmth, and comfort. So whip up a batch today, put your feet up, and dig in. It's medicine for whatever ails you. This low-fat, low-sodium version makes the most of wholesome chicken, toothsome noodles, and tender veggies. Add or omit vegetables and seasonings depending upon what you have on hand.

1. Combine all the ingredients except noodles in a stockpot. Bring to a boil over high heat.

2. Once boiling, add the noodles, reduce heat to medium-low, and simmer 10 minutes.

3. Remove from heat. Ladle soup into bowls and serve immediately.

**Per Serving (1½ cups)**

Calories: 291

Fat: 5 grams

Protein: 33 grams

Sodium: 167 milligrams

Fiber: 2 grams

Carbohydrates: 26 grams

Sugar: 2 grams

# Tofu Soup

**Prep Time:** 10 minutes
**Cook Time:** 5 minutes
**Total Time:** 15 minutes
**Serves 8**

## INGREDIENTS

8 cups low-sodium vegetable broth

8 cloves garlic, minced

3 medium carrots, diced

4 ounces mushrooms, sliced

6 scallions, sliced, divided

1-inch piece fresh ginger, minced

¼–½ teaspoon freshly ground white pepper

1 pound extra-firm tofu, cubed

### Ginger Facts

Ginger, also called gingerroot, has been used for hundreds of years as a natural remedy for many ailments, particularly nausea. It can be eaten raw, cooked, or ground, and adds a spicy, distinctive flavor to both sweet and savory dishes. Ginger contains antioxidants and anti-inflammatory compounds believed to inhibit cancer and cardiovascular disease.

This low-sodium soup is a natural cure-all. Tasty tofu cubes and vegetables are bathed in a light broth with a slightly spicy after-kick. For added heft, stir in some cooked soba wheat noodles or whole-grain angel hair pasta. If you have any dried nori (or other seaweed) in the cabinet, tear a sheet into pieces and add to the broth for some extra flavor.

1. Pour the broth into a stockpot. Add all of the ingredients except for the tofu and last 2 scallions. Bring to a boil over high heat.

2. Once boiling, add the tofu. Reduce heat to low, cover, and simmer for 5 minutes.

3. Remove from heat, ladle soup into bowls, and garnish with the remaining sliced scallions. Serve immediately.

**Per Serving (1½ cups)**

| | |
|---|---|
| Calories: 91 | Fiber: 2 grams |
| Fat: 3 grams | Carbohydrates: 8 grams |
| Protein: 6 grams | Sugar: 1 gram |
| Sodium: 153 milligrams | |

# Red Bean Stew with Spinach and Potatoes

**Prep Time:** 5 minutes
**Cook Time:** 25 minutes
**Total Time:** 30 minutes
**Serves 4**

## INGREDIENTS

1 tablespoon olive oil

1 medium onion, diced

8 cloves garlic, minced

1 medium stalk celery, diced

4 cups low-sodium vegetable broth

1 (15-ounce) can no-salt-added kidney beans, drained

3 small/medium potatoes, diced small

2 medium carrots, diced

2 teaspoons all-purpose salt-free seasoning

1 teaspoon dried basil

½ teaspoon dried thyme

Freshly ground black pepper, to taste

6 ounces fresh baby spinach

Juice of 1 lemon

Craving something warm and hearty, but pressed for time? This fabulous vegan stew is chock-full of the good stuff and comes together in just 30 minutes! The heft and bite of kidney beans works wonderfully in this recipe, but any type of cooked beans or legumes you have on hand will be fine. Serve over brown rice if desired.

1. Heat olive oil in a small stockpot over medium heat. Add onion, garlic, and celery and cook, stirring, 3 minutes. Add broth, beans, potatoes, carrots, and seasonings, raise heat to high, and bring to a boil. Once boiling, reduce heat to medium-low, cover, and simmer roughly 20 minutes, until beans are tender.

2. Remove from heat. Stir in the spinach until wilted fully. Squeeze in the lemon juice and stir to combine. Serve immediately.

**Per Serving (1½ cups)**

Calories: 285

Fat: 4 grams

Protein: 13 grams

Sodium: 212 milligrams

Fiber: 14 grams

Carbohydrates: 50 grams

Sugar: 3 grams

# Cheesy Potato Chowder

**Prep Time:** 4 minutes
**Cook Time:** 26 minutes
**Total Time:** 30 minutes
**Serves 6**

## INGREDIENTS

1 tablespoon olive oil

2 cups diced onion

1 cup diced celery

2 cloves garlic, minced

6 cups diced potato

4 cups low-sodium chicken broth

⅓ cup dry white wine

½ teaspoon dried thyme

¼ teaspoon ground rosemary

⅛ teaspoon dried basil

Freshly ground black pepper, to taste

1 cup shredded Swiss cheese

This creamy concoction of potatoes, chicken broth, and cheese will make a low-sodium soup fan of even the staunchest critic. If the potatoes are thin-skinned, leave the peel on for added nutrients and fiber. Be sure to dice the potatoes small to speed cooking time. White wine adds a lot of flavor, but if you avoid alcohol, substitute an equal amount of broth or a tablespoon or two of rice wine vinegar or white wine vinegar.

1. Heat olive oil in a stockpot over medium heat. Add onion, celery, and garlic and sauté for 5 minutes.

2. Add potato, broth, white wine, herbs, and black pepper, to taste.

3. Bring to a boil. Once boiling, reduce heat to low, cover, and simmer for 20 minutes.

4. Remove pot from heat. Using a blender or food processor, purée roughly half the soup. Return soup to pot and stir well to combine.

5. Add the shredded cheese and stir until melted.

6. Ladle the chowder into bowls and garnish with additional Swiss cheese, if desired. Serve hot.

**Per Serving (1½ cups)**

Calories: 252

Fat: 8 grams

Protein: 11 grams

Sodium: 94 milligrams

Fiber: 3 grams

Carbohydrates: 33 grams

Sugar: 3 grams

# Hearty Vegetable Beef Soup

**Prep Time:** 5 minutes
**Cook Time:** 25 minutes
**Total Time:** 30 minutes
**Serves 8**

### INGREDIENTS

1 pound lean ground beef

1 large onion, diced

3 medium carrots, sliced

3 medium stalks celery, sliced

6 cloves garlic, minced

1 (15-ounce) can no-salt-added diced tomatoes

1 (8-ounce) can no-salt-added tomato sauce

4 cups low-sodium beef broth

2 teaspoons dried Italian seasoning

Freshly ground black pepper, to taste

A great remedy for chilly winter weather, this no-nonsense recipe comes together in 30 minutes with ingredients you may already have on hand. To make an easy and equally delicious minestrone, omit the ground beef and substitute a can of chickpeas or kidney beans and a handful of cut green beans (fresh or frozen), instead. If you don't have beef broth, low-sodium vegetable or tomato juice works wonderfully.

1. Brown ground beef in a stockpot over medium heat. Once beef is cooked, carefully drain out any excess fat.

2. Add remaining ingredients to the pot, raise heat to high, and bring to a boil.

3. Once boiling, reduce heat to low, cover, and simmer for 20 minutes, stirring occasionally.

4. Remove from heat and serve immediately.

**Per Serving (1½ cups)**
Calories: 121
Fat: 3 grams
Protein: 13 grams
Sodium: 85 milligrams

Fiber: 2 grams
Carbohydrates: 11 grams
Sugar: 5 grams

# Mushroom Soup with Orzo

**Prep Time:** 7 minutes
**Cook Time:** 23 minutes
**Total Time:** 30 minutes
**Serves 6**

## INGREDIENTS

24 ounces fresh mushrooms

1 teaspoon olive oil

1 medium onion, diced

1 medium stalk celery, diced

6 cloves garlic, minced

6 cups low-sodium chicken or vegetable broth

½ teaspoon dried rosemary, crumbled

½ teaspoon dried sage, crumbled

½ teaspoon dried thyme

Freshly ground black pepper, to taste

⅔ cup dry orzo pasta

A warming dish for a nippy day, this soup is filled with the earthy flavors of mushrooms and garlic. Made from semolina flour, a type of wheat flour, orzo is a small, oval-shaped pasta with an appearance similar to rice. For a gluten-free alternative, try substituting cooked brown rice or quinoa for the orzo.

1. Clean the mushrooms. Slice half of them; chop the rest.

2. Heat olive oil in a stockpot over medium heat. Add the onion, celery, garlic, and mushrooms and sauté for 3 minutes.

3. Add the broth and seasonings, raise heat to high, and bring to a boil.

4. Once boiling, reduce heat to low, add the orzo, and stir well. Cover the pot and simmer 20 minutes.

5. Remove from heat and serve.

**Per Serving (1½ cups)**

Calories: 138

Fat: 3 grams

Protein: 10 grams

Sodium: 75 milligrams

Fiber: 2 grams

Carbohydrates: 21 grams

Sugar: 3 grams

# Summer Vegetable Stew

**Prep Time:** 5 minutes
**Cook Time:** 25 minutes
**Total Time:** 30 minutes
**Serves 6**

## INGREDIENTS

2 teaspoons olive oil

1 medium onion, diced

4 cloves garlic, minced

1 small/medium eggplant, peeled and diced

2 small yellow squash, diced

2 small zucchini, diced

6 small tomatoes, diced

2 (8-ounce) cans no-salt-added tomato sauce

1 cup red wine

1 teaspoon dried basil

1 teaspoon dried marjoram

¾ teaspoon freshly ground black pepper

½ teaspoon dried oregano

¼ teaspoon dried savory

This flavorful dish is light enough for the hottest of days, yet hearty enough to satisfy. Pair it with Soft and Crusty No-Rise Sandwich Rolls (see recipe in this chapter) for a lovely meal. A large 28-ounce can of salt-free diced tomatoes may be substituted for fresh when making this out of season. The red wine adds a lot of flavor, but if you'd like to forgo the alcohol, you can use a few tablespoons of balsamic vinegar in its place.

1. Heat olive oil in a large sauté pan over medium heat. Add all of the vegetables and cook, stirring, for 5 minutes.

2. Add tomato sauce, wine, and seasonings and stir to combine.

3. Cover pan and simmer for 20 minutes, stirring occasionally. Serve warm or at room temperature.

**Per Serving (1½ cups)**

Calories: 122

Fat: 2 grams

Protein: 2 grams

Sodium: 16 milligrams

Fiber: 3 grams

Carbohydrates: 17 grams

Sugar: 9 grams

# Easy Wonton Soup

Prep Time: 5 minutes
Cook Time: 15 minutes
Total Time: 20 minutes
Serves 8

## INGREDIENTS

½ pound lean ground pork

1 tablespoon minced fresh ginger

4 cloves garlic, minced

8 cups low-sodium chicken broth

2 cups sliced fresh mushrooms

6 ounces dry whole-grain yolk-free egg noodles

¼ teaspoon ground white pepper

4 scallions, sliced

This low-sodium soup mimics classic wonton so much, you'll be hard-pressed to tell the difference. Add your choice of fresh mushrooms: from basic white button or baby bella, to oyster or shiitake. For a vegetarian version, use vegetable broth and omit the ground pork. Ground white pepper adds a spicy kick to the soup, but if you don't have it handy, freshly ground black pepper will work just fine.

1. Place a stockpot over medium heat. Add the ground pork, ginger, and garlic and sauté for 5 minutes. Drain any excess fat, then return to stovetop.

2. Add the broth and bring to a boil. Once boiling, stir in the mushrooms, noodles, and white pepper. Cover and simmer for 10 minutes.

3. Remove pot from heat. Stir in the scallions and serve immediately.

**Per Serving (1½ cups)**

Calories: 143

Fat: 4 grams

Protein: 12 grams

Sodium: 90 milligrams

Fiber: 1 gram

Carbohydrates: 14 grams

Sugar: 1 gram

# Kale Soup with Lemon and Tuna

**Prep Time:** 5 minutes
**Cook Time:** 25 minutes
**Total Time:** 30 minutes
**Serves 4**

## INGREDIENTS

1 teaspoon olive oil

1 medium onion, minced

3 cloves garlic, minced

Juice of 2 fresh lemons

8 cups chopped fresh kale, thick stems removed

4 cups low-sodium chicken or vegetable broth

2 (5-ounce) cans no-salt-added tuna, in water

1 teaspoon salt-free herbes de Provence

1 teaspoon all-purpose salt-free seasoning

Freshly ground black pepper, to taste

The citrus kiss of this healthy soup brings sunshine to the darkest days. No-salt-added canned tuna adds protein and omega-3 fatty acids, but you can substitute another cooked fish or omit it entirely for a strictly vegetarian soup. Herbes de Provence is a classic blend of French herbs and is typically comprised of dried basil, thyme, savory, fennel, and lavender. It gives a distinct flavor to many dishes, and is particularly well suited to grilled meats and seafood. Commercial blends of herbes de Provence are sold in supermarkets and online.

1. Heat olive oil in a stockpot over medium heat. Add the onion and garlic and sauté for 2 minutes.

2. Add lemon juice and kale and cook, stirring, until kale has wilted slightly, 2–3 minutes.

3. Add the remaining ingredients, stir, and cover. Raise heat to high and bring to a boil. Once boiling, reduce heat to low and simmer for 20 minutes.

4. Remove from heat and serve immediately.

**Per Serving (1½ cups)**
Calories: 205
Fat: 4 grams
Protein: 27 grams
Sodium: 166 milligrams

Fiber: 3 grams
Carbohydrates: 18 grams
Sugar: 1 gram

# Sweet Potato and Chickpea Soup

Prep Time: 5 minutes
Cook Time: 20 minutes
Total Time: 25 minutes
Serves 4

## INGREDIENTS

1 (15-ounce) can no-salt-added chickpeas (also called garbanzo beans), drained

1 teaspoon olive oil

1 small/medium onion, chopped

1 garlic clove, minced

1-inch piece fresh ginger, minced

1 teaspoon salt-free garam masala

½ teaspoon ground sweet paprika

⅛ teaspoon dried red pepper flakes

4 cups low-sodium chicken or vegetable broth

4 cups cubed sweet potato

½ cup sliced carrot

2 tablespoons chopped fresh cilantro, for garnish

The intoxicating aromas of India were the inspiration for this sensational soup. Serve hot, garnished with chopped fresh cilantro. Be sure to peel and dice the sweet potatoes to speed up cooking. Use vegetable broth for a strictly vegan soup or, for a meatier one-dish meal, add cubed tempeh or a cooked, diced chicken breast.

1. Drain and rinse the chickpeas and set aside.

2. Heat olive oil in a stockpot over medium heat. Add onion and garlic and sauté for 2 minutes.

3. Add the ginger and spices and cook, stirring, for 30 seconds.

4. Add the broth and stir to combine. Add the sweet potatoes, carrots, and chickpeas and stir well.

5. Raise heat to high and bring to a boil. Once boiling, cover the pot, reduce heat to medium-low, and simmer for 15–18 minutes or until tender, stirring occasionally.

6. Remove from heat. Ladle into bowls, garnish with the fresh cilantro, and serve immediately.

**Per Serving (1½ cups)**
Calories: 348
Fat: 5 grams
Protein: 16 grams
Sodium: 163 milligrams

Fiber: 10 grams
Carbohydrates: 60 grams
Sugar: 18 grams

# Apple Butternut Soup

**Prep Time:** 10 minutes
**Cook Time:** 20 minutes
**Total Time:** 30 minutes
**Serves 6**

## INGREDIENTS

6 cups diced butternut squash

2 cups diced apple

6 cups water

2 cups unsweetened apple juice

½ teaspoon ground cinnamon

⅛ teaspoon ground allspice

### An Apple a Day

Apples are one of the most widely consumed fruits in the world. They can be eaten raw, cooked, dried, juiced, or fermented, without diminishing their nutritional value. To get the most of your apples, buy organic, wash them, and consume along with the skin, which provides added nutrients and fiber. Apples contain vitamins C and K as well as flavonoids, substances believed to prevent cancer.

Apples draw out the natural sweetness of butternut squash, delivering a smooth and irresistible fat-free soup. Although this soup is delicious year round, the flavors and color make it a particularly beautiful addition to a low-sodium Thanksgiving meal. Any type of apple works well here, from sweet to tart. Experiment with different varieties to find the kinds you like best.

1. Place diced squash and apple into a stockpot, add the water and apple juice, and bring to a boil over high heat. Once boiling, reduce heat to medium-low, cover, and simmer until tender, roughly 20 minutes.

2. Remove from heat. Add spices and stir to combine. Purée in a blender or food processor.

3. Serve warm.

**Per Serving (1 cup)**
Calories: 150
Fat: 0 grams
Protein: 3 grams
Sodium: 8 milligrams

Fiber: 1 gram
Carbohydrates: 38 grams
Sugar: 11 grams

# Black Bean Vegetable Soup

**Prep Time:** 5 minutes
**Cook Time:** 25 minutes
**Total Time:** 30 minutes
**Serves 4**

## INGREDIENTS

2½ cups low-sodium vegetable broth, divided

1 small red onion, diced

3 cloves garlic, minced

1 small carrot, diced

1 small stalk celery, diced

1 small sweet potato, diced

1 (15-ounce) can no-salt-added diced tomatoes

1 (15-ounce) can no-salt-added black beans

¼ cup red wine

1 tablespoon no-salt-added tomato paste

1½ teaspoons ground cumin

1 teaspoon dried oregano

½ teaspoon ground coriander

¼ teaspoon dried red pepper flakes

Freshly ground black pepper, to taste

2 tablespoons chopped fresh cilantro

Thick and hearty with a deep, rich taste, this low-fat vegetarian soup is ready in just 30 minutes. Don't drain the canned tomatoes or beans since the liquid will become part of the flavorful stock. The red wine adds distinct flavor, but, if you're avoiding alcohol, you can substitute a tablespoon or two of balsamic or red wine vinegar instead.

1. Place a stockpot over medium heat. Add ¼ cup of the vegetable broth, as well as the onion and garlic, and sauté for 2 minutes.

2. Add another ¼ cup broth, plus the carrot, celery, sweet potato, and tomatoes (including liquid) and sauté for 3 minutes.

3. Add remaining ingredients, except cilantro. Bring to a boil, cover, and reduce to a simmer for 15–20 minutes, until veggies are tender.

4. Remove from heat, stir in the cilantro, and serve immediately.

**Per Serving (1½ cups)**
Calories: 233
Fat: 2 grams
Protein: 10 grams
Sodium: 88 milligrams
Fiber: 8 grams
Carbohydrates: 41 grams
Sugar: 6 grams

# Chicken Soup with Jalapeño and Lime

**Prep Time:** 10 minutes
**Cook Time:** 15 minutes
**Total Time:** 25 minutes
**Serves 8**

## INGREDIENTS

2 cups cooked, shredded chicken

1 medium red onion, diced

3 cloves garlic, minced

2 medium carrots, sliced

1 medium stalk celery, sliced

1 medium red bell pepper, diced

1 jalapeño pepper, minced

1 (15-ounce) can no-salt-added diced tomatoes

Juice of 2 fresh limes

8 cups low-sodium chicken broth

1 teaspoon ground cumin

½ teaspoon ground coriander

¼ teaspoon dried oregano

Freshly ground black pepper, to taste

2 tablespoons chopped fresh cilantro

1 fresh lime, cut into wedges

Set your taste buds abuzz with the zing of fresh lime! This low-sodium soup is brimming with flavor, yet nearly fat-free. For added heft, ladle soup over bowls of cooked brown or wild rice, egg noodles, or quinoa. To reduce the amount of "heat," remove the seeds from the jalapeño. If you are particularly sensitive, wear disposable gloves while mincing the pepper, and be sure not to touch your face, nose, or eyes.

1. Place all the ingredients except cilantro and lime wedges into a stockpot and bring to a boil over high heat.

2. Once boiling, reduce heat to low, cover, and simmer for 15 minutes.

3. Remove from heat, ladle into bowls, and garnish with chopped cilantro and lime wedges. Serve immediately.

**Per Serving (1½ cups)**

| | |
|---|---|
| Calories: 118 | Fiber: 1 gram |
| Fat: 2 grams | Carbohydrates: 9 grams |
| Protein: 6 grams | Sugar: 3 grams |
| Sodium: 111 milligrams | |

# CHAPTER 5

# Snacks and Drinks

Holy Guacamole

Fat-Free Black Bean Dip

Garlic Lovers Hummus

Mango Salsa

Sour Cream and Onion Dip

Chewy Granola Bars

Whole-Grain Crackers

Homemade Soft Pretzels

Cheesy Seasoned Popcorn

Seasoned Sesame Kale Chips

Sweet Potato Crisps

Ginger Lemonade

Cranberry Limeade

Pumpkin Coconut Smoothies

Super Green Smoothies

Orange Creamsicle Smoothies

Chocolate-Covered Banana Milkshakes

Maple Mocha Frappe

Thin Mint Cocoa

Sweet Milky Chai Tea

# Holy Guacamole

**Prep Time:** 5 minutes
**Cook Time:** 0 minutes
**Total Time:** 5 minutes
**Yields 1 cup (8 servings)**

## INGREDIENTS

1 ripe avocado

1 small ripe tomato, chopped

Juice of 1 fresh lime

2 cloves garlic, minced

1 tablespoon chopped fresh cilantro

½ teaspoon ground cumin

Pinch ground cayenne pepper

All-purpose salt-free seasoning, to taste

Ripe avocados are one my favorite things to prepare. From their magnificent color, to their intoxicating tactile experience—the leather-like armor giving way to perfect smoothness—they're like an allegory of the human soul. Vibrant in color and flavor, this simple dip makes any meal more special. Serve with everything from chips to tacos to rice and beans. Guacamole is best consumed fresh, so serve the same day.

1. Peel, pit, and dice the avocado, then place in a deep bowl and mash with a fork until it's as smooth or coarse as desired.

2. Add remaining ingredients and mix well.

3. Serve immediately or cover and chill before serving.

**Per Serving (2 tablespoons)**

| | |
|---|---|
| Calories: 45 | Fiber: 2 grams |
| Fat: 3 grams | Carbohydrates: 3 grams |
| Protein: 0 grams | Sugar: 0 grams |
| Sodium: 3 milligrams | |

# Fat-Free Black Bean Dip

**Prep Time:** 2 minutes
**Cook Time:** 0 minutes
**Total Time:** 2 minutes
**Yields 1½ cups (12 servings)**

## INGREDIENTS

1 (15-ounce) can no-salt-added black beans

¼ cup fresh cilantro

2 cloves garlic

Juice of 1 fresh lime

1½ teaspoons ground cumin

½ teaspoon ground coriander

⅛ teaspoon ground cayenne

All-purpose salt-free seasoning, to taste

Freshly ground black pepper, to taste

### Squeeze Your Citrus

To get the most out of citrus fruit, give it a squeeze! Before juicing, roll citrus on the counter, pressing down firmly with your hands. The pressure will allow more of the juice to be extracted and it'll make your hands smell great, too! Another tip: When citrus gets old, it often dries out inside. Microwave older fruit for 15 seconds to get the most juice from your squeeze.

Completely guilt-free and so good! A chorus line of black beans, cilantro, and garlic with a zippy high kick of lime. Serve with fresh vegetables, unsalted tortilla chips, or as a filling or topping for burritos. If you can't find salt-free black beans, regular canned black beans will do. Just be sure to drain and rinse well to remove as much sodium as possible.

1. Drain black beans and rinse well.
2. Place all the ingredients in a food processor and pulse until smooth.
3. Serve immediately or cover and refrigerate until serving.

**Per Serving (2 tablespoons)**

Calories: 49
Fat: <1 gram
Protein: 3 grams
Sodium: 1 milligram

Fiber: 3 grams
Carbohydrates: 9 grams
Sugar: 0 grams

# Garlic Lovers Hummus

**Prep Time:** 2 minutes
**Cook Time:** 0 minutes
**Total Time:** 2 minutes
**Yields 1½ cups (12 servings)**

## INGREDIENTS

1 (15-ounce) can no-salt-added garbanzo beans (also called chickpeas)

3 tablespoons sesame tahini

3 tablespoons freshly squeezed lemon juice

2 tablespoons olive oil

4 cloves garlic

All-purpose salt-free seasoning, to taste

The ultimate vegetarian dip and sandwich filling. This version calls for tahini, a smooth sesame butter sold in many supermarkets and natural food stores. If you can't find it, try substituting low-sodium vegetable broth. For a milder flavor, reduce the amount of garlic, or for a spicier version, add a dash of hot sauce or some dried red pepper flakes to the mix.

1. Drain garbanzo beans and rinse well.

2. Place all the ingredients in a food processor and pulse until smooth.

3. Serve immediately or cover and refrigerate until serving.

**Per Serving (2 tablespoons)**

| | |
|---|---|
| Calories: 103 | Fiber: 3 grams |
| Fat: 5 grams | Carbohydrates: 11 grams |
| Protein: 4 grams | Sugar: 2 grams |
| Sodium: 7 milligrams | |

# Mango Salsa

Prep Time: 7 minutes
Cook Time: 0 minutes
Total Time: 7 minutes
Yields 2 cups (16 servings)

## INGREDIENTS

1 ripe mango, peeled and diced

1 small red bell pepper, chopped

2 cloves garlic, minced

1 jalapeño pepper, minced

Juice of 1 fresh lime

2 tablespoons chopped fresh cilantro

1 tablespoon apple cider vinegar

1 teaspoon agave nectar

1 teaspoon ground cumin

### Follow Your Nose

When selecting fresh mangoes, follow your nose. Sniff the stem end of the mango for clues to ripeness. Still in doubt? Let your fingers be your guide. Ripe mangoes will yield to gentle pressure, less ripe will give only a little, and unripe will remain hard. Select fruit with smooth, unblemished skin. And don't be fooled by the color of the peel; it has nothing to do with ripeness.

Ripe mangoes, garlic, lime, and cilantro flavor one of the most mouthwatering salsas ever. When mangoes are out of season, substitute an equal amount of fresh or canned pineapple chunks. Be creative with the recipe and try it out with other fruits like fresh strawberries, ripe peaches, and, yes, garden-ripe tomatoes.

1. Place all the ingredients in a bowl and stir well to combine.

2. Serve immediately or cover and refrigerate until ready to serve.

**Per Serving (2 tablespoons)**

| | |
|---|---|
| Calories: 16 | Fiber: 0 grams |
| Fat: 0 grams | Carbohydrates: 4 grams |
| Protein: 0 grams | Sugar: 3 grams |
| Sodium: 1 milligram | |

# Sour Cream and Onion Dip

**Prep Time:** 2 minutes
**Cook Time:** 5 minutes
**Total Time:** 7 minutes
**Yields 1 cup (16 servings)**

## INGREDIENTS

1 medium onion, diced
1 cup nonfat sour cream
1 teaspoon all-purpose salt-free seasoning
¼ teaspoon garlic powder

This rich, creamy, and guilt-free alternative to commercial dips is a terrific addition to baked potatoes, scrambled eggs, and fresh-cut veggies. The sautéed onion lends great flavor and texture to an otherwise smooth dip. If you're really pressed for time, feel free to substitute a tablespoon of onion powder instead.

1. Sauté the onion in a nonstick skillet over medium heat until soft and brown, roughly 5 minutes.

2. Place the remaining ingredients into a small mixing bowl. Add sautéed onion and stir well to combine.

3. Cover and refrigerate until serving.

**Per Serving (1 tablespoon)**
Calories: 23
Fat: 0 grams
Protein: 1 gram
Sodium: 42 milligrams
Fiber: 0 grams
Carbohydrates: 4 grams
Sugar: 0 grams

# Chewy Granola Bars

Prep Time: 5 minutes
Cook Time: 20 minutes
Total Time: 25 minutes
Yields 20 bars

## INGREDIENTS

3 cups quick oats

1 cup white whole-wheat flour

2 teaspoons sodium-free baking soda

1 teaspoon ground cinnamon

¼ teaspoon ground nutmeg

1½ cups unsweetened applesauce

¾ cup brown sugar

2 teaspoons pure vanilla extract

⅔ cup raisins or dried cranberries

These soft and chewy granola bars taste just like the ones you'd find in grocery stores, except they're fat-free and virtually sodium-free. Perfect for a quick energy boost, these bars are a guilt-free snack you can enjoy anytime and anywhere. Swap the dried fruit for chocolate chips or chopped nuts for a different variation. Adapted from WomenHeart's *All Heart Family Cookbook.*

1. Preheat oven to 350°F. Spray two 8-inch square baking pans lightly with oil and set aside.

2. Place the oats, flour, baking soda, cinnamon, and nutmeg into a mixing bowl and whisk well to combine.

3. Add the applesauce, brown sugar, and vanilla and mix well. Stir in the dried fruit. Divide the mixture evenly between the 2 prepared pans and smooth down. Place pans on the middle rack in oven and bake 20 minutes.

4. Remove pans from oven and place on wire rack to cool briefly. Cut each pan into 10 equal-sized bars. Carefully remove bars from pans and place on wire rack to cool. Serve immediately, store in an airtight container, or wrap individually and freeze.

**Per Serving (1 granola bar)**

Calories: 122
Fat: 1 gram
Protein: 2 grams
Sodium: 4 milligrams

Fiber: 2 grams
Carbohydrates: 27 grams
Sugar: 13 grams

# Whole-Grain Crackers

**Prep Time:** 20 minutes
**Cook Time:** 10 minutes
**Total Time:** 30 minutes
**Yields** 6½ dozen

## INGREDIENTS

1⅔ cups white whole-wheat flour

½ teaspoon sodium-free baking powder

1 tablespoon all-purpose salt-free seasoning

1 teaspoon ground rosemary

1 teaspoon garlic powder

½ cup low-fat milk

¼ cup grated Parmesan cheese

3 tablespoons olive oil

1 egg white

1–2 tablespoons water, if needed

These crisp salt-free crackers make super snacks. For a light and tasty meal, pair them with soup, sliced Swiss cheese, and crunchy grapes. To further reduce the fat in this recipe, swap the low-fat milk for skim, or the Parmesan cheese for nutritional yeast flakes. After baking, cool fully before storing in an airtight container to keep the crackers crisp.

1. Preheat oven to 400°F. Spray a baking sheet lightly with oil and set aside.

2. Place the flour, baking powder, and seasonings into a mixing bowl and whisk well to combine.

3. Add the milk, cheese, olive oil, and egg white and stir to make a stiff dough. Add 1–2 tablespoons of water if the dough is still a little too dry.

4. Turn the dough out onto a lightly floured surface and knead several minutes, until dough is smooth and intact. Roll out to roughly ⅛-inch thickness, but no thinner or the crackers will burn. Cut into 1½-inch squares and transfer to the prepared baking sheet.

5. Place baking sheet on middle rack in oven and bake 10 minutes. Remove from oven and place crackers on wire rack to cool. Once cool, store in an airtight container.

**Per Serving (6 crackers)**
Calories: 95
Fat: 4 grams
Protein: 3 grams
Sodium: 38 milligrams

Fiber: 2 grams
Carbohydrates: 12 grams
Sugar: 1 gram

# Homemade Soft Pretzels

**Prep Time:** 15 minutes
**Cook Time:** 15 minutes
**Total Time:** 30 minutes
**Yields 10**

## INGREDIENTS

4½ teaspoons dry active yeast

1½ cups warm water

2 tablespoons honey

3 cups unbleached all-purpose flour

1 cup white whole-wheat flour

2 tablespoons all-purpose salt-free seasoning

1 egg, beaten (for brushing)

Delicious, hot-from-the-oven, soft pretzels are easier to make than you might think. This low-fat, low-sodium version substitutes all-purpose salt-free seasoning for coarse salt. After baking, spray lightly with oil and sprinkle with nutritional yeast or another seasoning. Or enjoy them plain or served with salt-free mustard. Feel free to play around with this basic recipe to make it your own. Try adding cinnamon and sugar to create a sweet version, or add your favorite lean meat to make it even more savory.

1. Preheat oven to 425°F. Take out a large baking sheet and set aside.

2. Place the yeast into a large mixing bowl. Add water, honey, flours, and seasoning and stir to combine. Turn dough out onto a lightly floured surface and knead 5 minutes.

3. Divide dough into 10 equal pieces. Roll each piece into a long snake-like tube, then twist to form a pretzel. Place pretzels onto the baking sheet an inch or two apart and brush lightly with the beaten egg.

4. Place baking sheet on middle rack in oven and bake 15 minutes, until golden brown. Remove from oven and place pretzels on a wire rack to cool.

**Per Serving (1 pretzel)**
Calories: 200
Fat: 1 gram
Protein: 6 grams
Sodium: 8 milligrams

Fiber: 3 grams
Carbohydrates: 41 grams
Sugar: 4 grams

# Cheesy Seasoned Popcorn

**Prep Time:** 2 minutes
**Cook Time:** 5 minutes
**Total Time:** 7 minutes
**Yields 10 cups**

## INGREDIENTS

2 tablespoons nutritional yeast flakes

1½ teaspoons dried dill

1 teaspoon dried parsley

¾ teaspoon garlic powder

¾ teaspoon onion powder

½ teaspoon ground sweet paprika

¼ teaspoon dried thyme

¼ teaspoon freshly ground black pepper

½ cup popcorn kernels

2 teaspoons olive oil

I've had a love/hate relationship with popcorn since being diagnosed with Meniere's disease. Basically, I love it, but hate the fact that I can't sprinkle it with salt. This popcorn recipe has changed all that. I've made (and varied) it several times with delicious success. Think of this as a suggestion; something to try and adapt as desired. This seasoned popcorn will satisfy salty snack cravings anytime.

1. Measure the nutritional yeast, dill, parsley, garlic powder, onion powder, paprika, thyme, and black pepper into a small bowl and stir well to combine. Set aside.

2. Place popcorn kernels into an air popper. Place a stockpot beneath the popcorn dispenser, turn appliance on, and wait until kernels have popped. Turn off popper and set aside.

3. Drizzle the olive oil over the popcorn and toss well to coat. Once popcorn is thoroughly coated with oil, sprinkle with the seasoning mixture and stir vigorously for several minutes until completely coated.

4. Serve immediately or store in an airtight container until serving.

**Per Serving (1 cup)**
Calories: 55
Fat: 1 gram
Protein: 2 grams
Sodium: 2 milligrams

Fiber: 2 grams
Carbohydrates: 8 grams
Sugar: <1 gram

# Seasoned Sesame Kale Chips

**Prep Time:** 5 minutes
**Cook Time:** 12 minutes
**Total Time:** 17 minutes
**Serves 4**

## INGREDIENTS

1 bunch fresh kale

Spray oil

2½ teaspoons Bragg Organic Sea Kelp Delight Seasoning

2 teaspoons toasted sesame seeds

### What Is Kelp?

Kelp is a type of harvested seaweed. It's naturally low in sodium with a pronounced salty taste, making it an excellent salt substitute. Kelp is low in fat and calories, aids metabolism through its high concentration of iodine, and is a great source of Vitamin K and folate. Kelp is sold in dried form, either alone or as part of a seasoning blend. Maine Coast Sea Vegetables Organic Kelp Granules and Bragg Organic Sea Kelp Delight Seasoning are two such products and both are sold in select stores and online.

Light as air, crisp, and addictive, these chips get their salty taste from low-sodium kelp seasoning. If you don't like the flavor of seaweed, or can't find it, any favorite salt-free seasoning will do. Before baking, sprinkle with nutritional yeast flakes for a yummy, cheesy taste. Or add some red pepper flakes to the mix for a spicy variation.

1. Preheat oven to 325°F. Lightly spray a baking sheet with oil and set aside.

2. Wash kale and pat dry thoroughly with paper towel. Remove leaves from the tough stalks, cut or tear into pieces, and arrange in a single layer on the baking sheet.

3. Spray lightly with oil and sprinkle with seasoning and sesame seeds.

4. Place baking sheet on middle rack in oven and bake 12 minutes. Remove from oven and transfer chips to a sheet of waxed paper or foil to cool. Repeat process with remaining ingredients.

5. Store in an airtight container.

**Per Serving (1 cup)**

| | |
|---|---|
| Calories: 41 | Fiber: 2 grams |
| Fat: 1 gram | Carbohydrates: 7 grams |
| Protein: 2 grams | Sugar: 0 grams |
| Sodium: 77 milligrams | |

# Sweet Potato Crisps

**Prep Time:** 7 minutes
**Cook Time:** 16 minutes
**Total Time:** 23 minutes
**Serves 2**

## INGREDIENTS

1 medium sweet potato, scrubbed well
2 teaspoons olive oil
½ teaspoon ground sweet paprika

Love store-bought sweet potato chips? This homemade version is so good you may never buy them again. To save time, slice the sweet potatoes using a food processor or handheld mandolin. If you're using a knife, just be sure to cut the sweet potatoes as thinly and uniformly as possible. Adapted from Chow.com.

1. Position 2 oven racks in the middle of the oven, one right over the other. Preheat oven to 350°F. Take out 2 baking sheets and set aside.

2. Slice the sweet potato into paper-thin rounds using a mandolin or very sharp knife.

3. Place slices into a mixing bowl, add the olive oil and paprika, and toss well to coat. Arrange the slices in a single layer on the baking sheets. Do not overlap.

4. Place the baking sheets on the middle 2 racks in the oven and bake 8 minutes. Switch the baking sheet positions and bake another 7–8 minutes, until the edges of the slices begin to curl and the centers are golden brown and dry to the touch.

5. Remove baking sheets from the oven and place on wire racks. Cool for a few minutes before transferring to a bowl. Serve immediately or store in an airtight container for up to 3 days.

**Per Serving (1 cup)**

| | |
|---|---|
| Calories: 93 | Fiber: 2 grams |
| Fat: 4 grams | Carbohydrates: 12 grams |
| Protein: 1 gram | Sugar: 4 grams |
| Sodium: 21 milligrams | |

# Ginger Lemonade

**Prep Time:** 5 minutes
**Cook Time:** 0 minutes
**Total Time:** 5 minutes
Serves 4

## INGREDIENTS

¼ cup minced fresh ginger

Minced zest of 1 fresh lemon

1 cup freshly squeezed lemon juice

3 cups water

5 tablespoons sugar

There's nothing so refreshing on a hot day as a glass of ice-cold lemonade. Here, the spicy flavor and aroma of ginger adds depth, sophistication, and kick. If you have time, make this ahead and let it steep for several hours in the refrigerator. The flavors improve the longer they're allowed to sit. Don't have extra time? It's still fabulous!

1. Place the minced ginger and lemon zest into a small pitcher. Add the lemon juice, water, and sugar, and stir well to combine.

2. When ready to serve, fill 4 tall glasses with ice, pour lemonade over the ice, and serve. Flavors will develop more fully the longer the lemonade is allowed to steep.

**Per Serving (1 cup)**
Calories: 75
Fat: 0 grams
Protein: 0 grams
Sodium: 8 milligrams

Fiber: 0 grams
Carbohydrates: 21 grams
Sugar: 17 grams

# Cranberry Limeade

**Prep Time:** 5 minutes
**Cook Time:** 0 minutes
**Total Time:** 5 minutes
**Serves 6**

## INGREDIENTS

1 cup freshly squeezed lime juice

Grated zest of 1 fresh lime

3 cups water

1 cup cranberry juice (100% juice blend)

¼ cup sugar

### Cranberry Facts

Cranberries contain numerous anti-oxidants, high levels of vitamin C, and have even been reported to inhibit cancer. But perhaps what they're best known for is their ability to protect against urinary tract infections. A substance within the cranberry is thought to prevent bacteria from adhering to the bladder wall, thus preventing attack.

Cranberry juice and lime are a match made in heaven. Sweet, tart, and tangy, it's best served ice-cold. Don't have lime juice? Try lemon or orange instead. For an extra-pretty party-worthy presentation, serve the limeade in a glass pitcher with sliced fruit rounds and ice. For adult beverages, add a shot of vodka to the mix.

1. Measure all the ingredients into a large pitcher and stir well to combine.

2. Serve immediately or refrigerate until ready to serve.

**Per Serving (1 cup)**

Calories: 62
Fat: 0 grams
Protein: 0 grams
Sodium: 6 milligrams

Fiber: 0 grams
Carbohydrates: 17 grams
Sugar: 14 grams

# Pumpkin Coconut Smoothies

**Prep Time:** 2 minutes
**Cook Time:** 0 minutes
**Total Time:** 2 minutes
**Serves 3**

## INGREDIENTS

½ cup pumpkin purée
1 cup light coconut milk
½ cup low-fat vanilla yogurt
1 tablespoon agave nectar

Thick, creamy, and absolutely delicious, these pumpkin smoothies are a great alternative to the high-fat frozen treats sold each fall. Plus, thanks to canned pumpkin, you can enjoy them year round! For an extra-special treat, top with low-fat whipped cream and sprinkle with ground cinnamon or chocolate shavings.

1. Measure all ingredients into a blender or food processor and pulse until smooth.

2. Serve immediately.

**Per Serving (⅔ cup)**
Calories: 121
Fat: 6 grams
Protein: 2 grams
Sodium: 36 milligrams

Fiber: 1 gram
Carbohydrates: 10 grams
Sugar: 8 grams

# Super Green Smoothies

**Prep Time:** 5 minutes
**Cook Time:** 0 minutes
**Total Time:** 5 minutes
**Serves 2**

## INGREDIENTS

1 cup baby spinach

1 ripe kiwi fruit

1 ripe banana

1 cup mango juice

½ cup nonfat vanilla yogurt

Tender baby spinach gives these smoothies their bright color and nutrient boost. The sweet and fruity flavor hides the spinach so well that you'd never guess it's in there! Feel free to substitute baby kale for the spinach, pineapple or another low-sodium juice blend for the mango, or fruit yogurt for the vanilla yogurt. For a vegan version, use nondairy yogurt instead.

1. Place spinach into a blender or food processor and purée.

2. Add the kiwi and banana and purée again.

3. Add remaining ingredients and pulse until smooth and creamy.

4. Serve immediately.

**Per Serving (1⅓ cup)**
Calories: 196
Fat: 0 grams
Protein: 4 grams
Sodium: 40 milligrams

Fiber: 4 grams
Carbohydrates: 40 grams
Sugar: 26 grams

# Orange Creamsicle Smoothies

**Prep Time:** 2 minutes
**Cook Time:** 0 minutes
**Total Time:** 2 minutes
**Serves 2**

## INGREDIENTS

1 large navel orange
1 cup vanilla nondairy milk

A healthy, low-fat vegan shake with a deliciously decadent taste. These creamsicle smoothies are just like the frozen treats, but better. When peeling the orange, be sure to remove as much of the bitter white pith as possible. Or for speed, substitute a couple of easy-peeling clementines for the navel orange whenever they're in season.

1. Peel orange, removing as much of the white pith as possible.

2. Segment orange and purée in blender or food processor. Add nondairy milk and pulse until smooth.

3. Serve immediately.

**Per Serving (¾ cup)**

| | |
|---|---|
| Calories: 84 | Fiber: 2 grams |
| Fat: 2 grams | Carbohydrates: 14 grams |
| Protein: 3 grams | Sugar: 10 grams |
| Sodium: 57 milligrams | |

# Chocolate-Covered Banana Milkshakes

**Prep Time:** 2 minutes
**Cook Time:** 0 minutes
**Total Time:** 2 minutes
Serves 2

## INGREDIENTS

1 ripe banana

1 cup vanilla nonfat frozen yogurt

1 tablespoon unsweetened cocoa powder

1 cup low-fat milk

### Blenders versus Food Processors

Can't decide which appliance to invest in? Think about long-term use. For drinks, a blender may be the best choice. But if you're looking to purée and chop as well as blend, a food processor may be a better option. Also consider how often you'll be using the appliance. For light use, an inexpensive model works well. For heavy use, invest in a large-capacity appliance with a strong motor and warranty. Do research and read reviews before deciding.

Decadent taste with zero guilt! These low-fat shakes are a healthy and satisfying alternative to traditional ice cream parlor fare. For extra-rich chocolate flavor, use chocolate nonfat frozen yogurt instead. Or for a super, low-sodium, banana split shake, add some fresh or frozen strawberries, top with low-fat whipped cream, sprinkles, and a cherry!

1. Place banana into a blender or food processor and purée.

2. Add remaining ingredients and pulse until smooth.

3. Serve immediately.

**Per Serving (1⅓ cups)**

| | |
|---|---|
| Calories: 209 | Fiber: 2 grams |
| Fat: 2 grams | Carbohydrates: 42 grams |
| Protein: 9 grams | Sugar: 32 grams |
| Sodium: 124 milligrams | |

# Maple Mocha Frappe

**Prep Time:** 2 minutes
**Cook Time:** 0 minutes
**Total Time:** 2 minutes
Serves 2

## INGREDIENTS

1 small ripe banana

½ cup brewed coffee

½ cup low-fat milk

1 cup low-fat vanilla yogurt

1 tablespoon unsweetened cocoa powder

2 tablespoons pure maple syrup

A creamy concoction of coffee, cocoa, milk, and maple syrup, this drink is perfect for breakfast or as an anytime pick-me-up. Just keep in mind that the stronger the coffee, the more flavor it lends to the drink. For less of a jolt, feel free to use decaffeinated coffee. Or for more coffee flavor, use low-fat coffee yogurt.

1. Place the banana in a blender or food processor and purée.

2. Add the remaining ingredients and pulse until smooth and creamy.

3. Serve immediately.

**Per Serving (1 cup)**
Calories: 206
Fat: 2 grams
Protein: 6 grams
Sodium: 116 milligrams

Fiber: 2 grams
Carbohydrates: 38 grams
Sugar: 30 grams

# Thin Mint Cocoa

**Prep Time:** 2 minutes
**Cook Time:** 5 minutes
**Total Time:** 7 minutes
Serves 4

### INGREDIENTS

3½ cups vanilla nondairy milk

¼ cup unsweetened cocoa powder

¼ cup light brown sugar

¼ teaspoon pure peppermint extract

I've made many variations of hot chocolate over the years, but this one is by far my favorite. This fabulous recipe is truly heaven in a cocoa: super simple and totally sublime. Like a liquid form of the famous Girl Scout cookie, but with much less guilt, this healthy vegan version of the traditional treat will make mouths and tummies tingle.

1. Measure nondairy milk into a saucepan and place over medium-high heat.

2. Once milk begins to steam, roughly 3–5 minutes, add cocoa and brown sugar, and whisk well to combine.

3. Remove from heat. Stir in the peppermint extract and serve immediately.

**Per Serving (1 cup)**

Calories: 134

Fat: 4 grams

Protein: 7 grams

Sodium: 83 milligrams

Fiber: 3 grams

Carbohydrates: 20 grams

Sugar: 14 grams

# Sweet Milky Chai Tea

**Prep Time:** 3 minutes
**Cook Time:** 5 minutes
**Total Time:** 8 minutes
**Serves 6**

## INGREDIENTS

6 tea bags

5 cups water

1 cup low-fat milk

½ cup honey

1 teaspoon pure vanilla extract

¼ teaspoon ground cloves

¼ teaspoon ground ginger

⅛ teaspoon ground allspice

⅛ teaspoon ground cardamom

⅛ teaspoon ground cinnamon

Years ago, I had the pleasure of attending an Indian wedding and it was an experience I'll never forget. With over 300 guests, the post-ceremony reception—which included pitcher after pitcher of sweet milky chai tea—was absolutely spectacular. This recipe is my humble attempt at re-creating that glorious day and one of the most delicious drinks I've ever had. Any standard black tea, with or without caffeine, will work fine here. For a refreshing hot weather treat, serve over ice.

1. Place all the ingredients into a saucepan and stir well to combine. When using conventional tea bags, carefully remove the tags and strings before placing in pot, but be sure to keep the bags sealed.

2. Heat over high until the contents begin to steam, but have not yet boiled, roughly 5 minutes. Turn off heat and let sit 1 minute.

3. Remove tea bags and ladle into a tea pot or mugs. Serve immediately.

**Per Serving (1 cup)**
Calories: 105
Fat: 0 grams
Protein: 1 gram
Sodium: 27 milligrams

Fiber: 0 grams
Carbohydrates: 25 grams
Sugar: 25 grams

# CHAPTER 6

# Appetizers and Side Dishes

Heavenly Deviled Eggs

Savory Stuffed Mushrooms

Baked Tofu with Tangy
Dipping Sauce

Coconut-Crusted Chicken with
Spicy-Sweet Dipping Sauce

Zucchini Sticks

Fat-Free Oven-Baked Fries

Baked Spinach and Pea Risotto

Roasted Root Veggies with
Orange and Thyme

Baked Apple Slices

Sweet and Savory Kale
with Tomatoes

Lemon Parmesan Rice
with Fresh Herbs

Braised Brussels Sprouts with
Apricots and Toasted Walnuts

Roasted Red Peppers

Whipped Sweet Potatoes

Quinoa Pilaf with
Mushrooms and Sage

Roasted Potatoes and Broccoli

Garlic Rosemary Mashed Potatoes

Carrots with Ginger,
Cilantro, and Lime

Southwestern Rice Pilaf

Curried Butternut Squash

Sautéed Spinach with
Onions and Garlic

Stir-Fried Cabbage and Noodles

Rice with Black Beans,
Mango, and Lime

Sun-Dried Tomato Couscous
with Pine Nuts and Basil

Garlic Steamed Squash

# Heavenly Deviled Eggs

**Prep Time:** 3 minutes
**Cook Time:** 12 minutes
**Total Time:** 15 minutes
**Serves 6**

## INGREDIENTS

6 large eggs

1 tablespoon nonfat sour cream

1 tablespoon water or low-sodium chicken broth

1 tablespoon finely chopped fresh chives

1 teaspoon no-salt-added prepared mustard

½ teaspoon dried herbes de Provence

Freshly ground black pepper, to taste

Ground sweet paprika, for garnish

### Snipping versus Slicing

When working with fresh herbs such as chives, it's often faster to snip them into small pieces using a pair of kitchen shears than it is to slice through them with a knife. A good pair of kitchen scissors can be purchased inexpensively, and the time you'll save is well worth the investment.

Creamy, tart, and addictive. To easily remove the shells from the cooked eggs, crack against a hard surface, then hold under cool running water. The peels should slide right off. Herbes de Provence is a blend of flavorful dried herbs that melds wonderfully with eggs. If you can't find it, use ½ teaspoon dried thyme instead.

1. Place eggs in a saucepan and add enough water to cover them by a couple inches. Bring to a boil over high heat, then lower heat slightly and boil 12 minutes.

2. Remove pan from heat, place in sink under cold running water, and let sit 1–2 minutes until eggs are cool enough to handle.

3. Peel eggs and slice in half lengthwise. Gently remove yolks and place in a small mixing bowl.

4. To the yolks, add the sour cream, water (or broth), chives, and mustard. Stir well to combine.

5. Crush the herbes de Provence in your hand and add to the mixture along with freshly ground black pepper, to taste. Mix until smooth.

6. Divide the yolk mixture evenly among the egg halves, filling neatly. Sprinkle with ground paprika and serve.

**Per Serving (2 deviled egg halves)**

| | |
|---|---|
| Calories: 79 | Fiber: 0 grams |
| Fat: 5 grams | Carbohydrates: 1 gram |
| Protein: 6 grams | Sugar: 0 grams |
| Sodium: 66 milligrams | |

# Savory Stuffed Mushrooms

**Prep Time:** 5 minutes
**Cook Time:** 15 minutes
**Total Time:** 20 minutes
**Serves 6**

## INGREDIENTS

16 ounces fresh mushrooms

2 tablespoons olive oil

½ cup salt-free bread crumbs

1 egg white

½ cup shredded Swiss cheese

4 cloves garlic

1 teaspoon dried Italian seasoning

½ teaspoon freshly ground black pepper

A lovely appetizer or side dish, these salt-free stuffed mushrooms have a crisp and tasty breading that's so good, they'll be gone before you know it. When removing the stems, be as gentle as possible! The goal is to keep the caps fully intact. Try mixing things up with a combination of white button mushrooms and baby bellas.

1. Preheat oven to 400°F. Spray a baking sheet lightly with oil and set aside.

2. Clean the mushrooms and gently remove stems, taking care to leave the caps intact. Set caps aside.

3. Place the mushroom stems in a food processor and add the remaining ingredients. Pulse several times to finely chop and combine the mixture.

4. Stuff each mushroom cap with the mixture, then place on the prepared baking sheet. Place sheet on middle rack in oven and bake 15 minutes. Remove from oven.

5. Mushrooms can be served warm or at room temperature.

**Per Serving (⅙ of the mushrooms)**

Calories: 124

Fat: 7 grams

Protein: 5 grams

Sodium: 30 milligrams

Fiber: 1 gram

Carbohydrates: 10 grams

Sugar: 1 gram

# Baked Tofu with Tangy Dipping Sauce

**Prep Time:** 10 minutes
**Cook Time:** 20 minutes
**Total Time:** 30 minutes
**Serves 8**

## INGREDIENTS

1 pound extra-firm tofu, drained

1 egg white

1 tablespoon water

½ cup salt-free bread crumbs

1 tablespoon dried parsley

1 teaspoon dried Italian seasoning

1 teaspoon ground sweet paprika

1 teaspoon onion powder

½ teaspoon garlic powder

½ teaspoon freshly ground black pepper

### DIPPING SAUCE

1 (8-ounce) can no-salt-added tomato sauce

1 tablespoon apple cider vinegar

1 tablespoon molasses

1 tablespoon honey

1 tablespoon dry ground mustard

½ teaspoon ground cumin

Pinch ground cayenne pepper

### What Is Tofu?

Tofu is made from soybeans in a process not unlike the making of cheese. Bean curds are separated from liquid and pressed into blocks. Tofu is sold in two main types. The first type, what many consider "regular" tofu, is sold in blocks submerged in liquid. It comes in silken, firm, and extra-firm varieties and must be kept refrigerated. The second type of tofu, which comes in shelf-stable packaging and does not need to be refrigerated, is silken style. It comes in varying levels of firmness, from silken to extra firm; all have a soft, smooth feel.

Bursting with flavor, these breaded, oven-fried cutlets will make a tofu lover out of you! Paired with a sweet, slightly spicy sauce, they're absolutely delicious. Be sure to press the tofu well to remove as much liquid as possible, but not so hard that you leave it mashed and mangled! If you're making this dish for larger parties, just double the quantity of tofu and sauce in the recipe.

1. Preheat oven to 425°F. Spray a baking sheet lightly with oil and set aside.

2. Gently press the drained tofu between paper towels to release excess liquid. Slice tofu in half lengthwise, then slice each half into 8 equal pieces. Set aside.

3. Beat the egg white and water in a shallow bowl until slightly foamy.

4. Place the bread crumbs into another bowl, add the seasonings (parsley through black pepper), and whisk well to combine.

5. Dip each piece of tofu in the egg white, then gently press in the bread crumbs to coat all sides. Place coated tofu cutlets on prepared baking sheet.

6. Place baking sheet on middle rack in oven and bake 10 minutes. Remove from oven, gently flip, and return to oven to bake another 10 minutes.

7. While tofu is baking, combine dipping sauce ingredients in a saucepan. Heat over medium-low heat, stirring frequently. Once mixture begins to

continued on next page

bubble, remove from heat and pour into a small serving bowl.

8. Remove tofu from oven and serve immediately with tangy dipping sauce.

**Per Serving (2 pieces of tofu and 2½ tablespoons sauce)**
Calories: 121                          Fiber: 2 grams
Fat: 3 grams                           Carbohydrates: 15 grams
Protein: 8 grams                       Sugar: 6 grams
Sodium: 15 milligrams

# Coconut-Crusted Chicken with Spicy-Sweet Dipping Sauce

**Prep Time:** 10 minutes
**Cook Time:** 20 minutes
**Total Time:** 30 minutes
**Serves 6**

## INGREDIENTS

4 boneless, skinless chicken thighs (or 8 ounces tempeh)

¼ cup unsweetened coconut

¼ cup salt-free bread crumbs

1 teaspoon garlic powder

¼ teaspoon freshly ground black pepper

1 egg white (or egg replacement powder)

### DIPPING SAUCE

2 tablespoons orange marmalade

1½ teaspoons unflavored rice vinegar

¼ teaspoon dried red pepper flakes

Deliciously crisp breading gives way to moist and tender chicken in this healthy alternative to coconut shrimp. A tasty vegan version can be created using tempeh and egg replacement powder. The sweet and tangy orange dipping sauce in this recipe gets a delicious kick from dried red pepper flakes. For more spice, add more pepper flakes or a dash of hot sauce.

1. Preheat oven to 425°F. Spray a baking sheet lightly with oil and set aside.

2. Wash the chicken and pat dry. Cut the chicken into 20 bite-sized pieces.

3. Measure the coconut, bread crumbs, garlic powder, and black pepper into a small mixing bowl and whisk well to combine. Set aside.

4. Place the egg white into a shallow bowl and beat well. (Or prepare egg replacement powder as directed.)

5. Dip each piece of chicken into the egg, then press into the bread crumbs to coat. Place on prepared baking sheet. Place sheet on middle rack in oven and bake 10 minutes.

6. Flip chicken and return to oven for another 10 minutes (only 5 minutes if using tempeh).

7. While chicken is baking, measure the marmalade, vinegar, and red pepper flakes into a small bowl and stir well to combine.

continued on next page

8. Remove baking sheet from oven and transfer chicken to a platter. Serve immediately along with the dipping sauce.

**Per Serving (3–4 pieces)**

Calories: 105

Fat: 4 grams

Protein: 7 grams

Sodium: 39 milligrams

Fiber: 1 gram

Carbohydrates: 10 grams

Sugar: 5 grams

# Zucchini Sticks

**Prep Time:** 10 minutes
**Cook Time:** 15 minutes
**Total Time:** 25 minutes
**Serves 6**

## INGREDIENTS

2 small/medium zucchini

1 egg white

1 tablespoon water

3 tablespoons salt-free bread crumbs

1 tablespoon grated Parmesan cheese

1 teaspoon dried Italian seasoning

½ teaspoon garlic powder

½ teaspoon onion powder

¼ teaspoon freshly ground black pepper

⅛ teaspoon ground sweet paprika

½ cup no-salt-added pasta sauce

Modeled after fried mozzarella, but without all the grease, these yummy zucchini sticks are crisp and golden on the outside and tender inside. Serve with jarred low-sodium pasta sauce for happy dipping. If you can't find commercial salt-free sauce locally, you can buy it online, make your own, or substitute the lowest-sodium sauce you can find.

1. Preheat oven to 450°F. Spray a baking sheet lightly with oil and set aside.

2. Trim ends off the zucchini, then cut in half. Quarter each of these halves, lengthwise, to make 16 (roughly) equal wedges.

3. Beat the egg white and water in a small shallow bowl. Set aside.

4. Place the bread crumbs, cheese, and seasonings into a small mixing bowl and whisk well to combine.

5. Dip each piece of zucchini in egg, then roll in bread crumbs. Place on baking sheet. Place baking sheet on middle rack in oven and bake for 15 minutes.

6. While zucchini is baking, gently warm pasta sauce on stovetop or in microwave. Pour into a small bowl and set aside.

7. Remove zucchini sticks from oven and serve immediately with the warm sauce.

**Per Serving (2–3 wedges)**
Calories: 39
Fat: 1 gram
Protein: 2 grams
Sodium: 28 milligrams

Fiber: 1 gram
Carbohydrates: 6 grams
Sugar: 2 grams

# Fat-Free Oven-Baked Fries

**Prep Time:** 5 minutes
**Cook Time:** 25 minutes
**Total Time:** 30 minutes
**Serves 4**

## INGREDIENTS

4 medium potatoes

1½ teaspoons all-purpose salt-free
seasoning

½ teaspoon freshly ground black pepper

Oven-baked fries are every bit as satisfying and delicious as those deep fried in oil, but they're even better because they're *fat-free!* This means you can have the best of both worlds: all the taste of your fast-food favorite without any of the guilt! Any kind of potato will work well in this recipe, but Red Bliss and Yukon gold potatoes are extra tasty when baked.

1. Preheat oven to 450°F. Spray a baking sheet lightly with oil and set aside.

2. Scrub potatoes and slice each into 8 equal wedges. Places wedges into a mixing bowl, add seasonings, and toss well to coat.

3. Arrange wedges cut side down on the prepared baking sheet. Place sheet on middle rack in oven and bake 15 minutes. Remove sheet from oven and gently flip wedges onto the second cut side. Return to middle rack in oven and bake another 10 minutes, until tender.

4. Remove baking sheet from oven. Serve immediately.

**Per Serving (8 potato wedges)**

Calories: 212

Fat: 0 grams

Protein: 4 grams

Sodium: 16 milligrams

Fiber: 4 grams

Carbohydrates: 48 grams

Sugar: 0 grams

# Baked Spinach and Pea Risotto

**Prep Time:** 5 minutes
**Cook Time:** 25 minutes
**Total Time:** 30 minutes
**Serves 6**

## INGREDIENTS

1 tablespoon unsalted butter

1 shallot, chopped

Freshly ground black pepper, to taste

½ cup dry white wine

3 cups low-sodium chicken broth

1 cup Arborio rice

1 cup frozen peas (thawed)

2 cups chopped fresh baby spinach

¼ cup grated Parmesan cheese

### Sodium in Frozen Vegetables

Many frozen vegetables are just that, frozen vegetables. But others contain things you don't want, like added salt and sauces. Even "plain" veggies may have been treated in such a way that elevates their sodium content. When selecting frozen vegetables, check nutrition facts carefully to ensure you're buying the vegetables you want, without anything else.

There's something magical about the combination of tastes and textures in this risotto. The wine, broth, and cheese lend so much flavor, and the creaminess keeps you coming back for more. If you're concerned about the sodium in the cheese, just eliminate it altogether—it will be just as delicious without it. If you're looking for a substitute for the wine, replace it with ¼ cup chicken broth mixed with 2–3 tablespoons of white wine vinegar. Adapted from *Real Simple*.

1. Preheat oven to 425°F.

2. Place a Dutch oven or similar lidded casserole pan on the stovetop over medium-high heat. Add the butter. Once melted, add the shallot and black pepper and sauté for 3 minutes.

3. Add the wine and cook, stirring, until almost evaporated, 2 minutes.

4. Add the broth and rice and bring to a boil.

5. Once boiling, cover the pot and transfer to the middle rack in the oven. Bake for 20 minutes, until rice is tender and creamy.

6. Remove from oven. Add the peas, spinach, and Parmesan and stir well to combine. If desired, season with additional ground black pepper, to taste. Serve immediately.

**Per Serving (⅔ cup)**

| | |
|---|---|
| Calories: 209 | Fiber: 1 gram |
| Fat: 4 grams | Carbohydrates: 32 grams |
| Protein: 7 grams | Sugar: 2 grams |
| Sodium: 110 milligrams | |

# Roasted Root Veggies with Orange and Thyme

**Prep Time:** 5 minutes
**Cook Time:** 25 minutes
**Total Time:** 30 minutes
**Serves 6**

## INGREDIENTS

3 medium carrots

3 medium parsnips

2 medium sweet potatoes

3 tablespoons freshly squeezed orange juice

1 tablespoon olive oil

1 teaspoon dried thyme

All-purpose salt-free seasoning, to taste

Freshly ground black pepper, to taste

A beautiful vegetable medley with bright color and taste. Cut the vegetables into uniformly sized pieces to ensure even cooking. Parsnips are great here for their subtle earthy sweetness and pale color, but if you can't find them or don't have any on hand, feel free to substitute 2 medium potatoes of any kind. You can either peel the veggies or simply scrub them well and retain the peels for added nutrients and fiber.

1. Preheat oven to 450°F. Take out a sided baking sheet and set aside.

2. Peel vegetables (or scrub well) and cut into ½-inch to 1-inch pieces. The smaller the chunks, the faster the cooking time. Place in a mixing bowl, add remaining ingredients, and toss well to coat.

3. Turn mixture out onto baking sheet and arrange vegetables in a single layer.

4. Place baking sheet on middle rack in oven and bake for 25 minutes.

5. Remove from oven and serve immediately.

**Per Serving (1 cup)**

| | |
|---|---|
| Calories: 123 | Fiber: 5 grams |
| Fat: 2 grams | Carbohydrates: 24 grams |
| Protein: 2 grams | Sugar: 7 grams |
| Sodium: 43 milligrams | |

# Baked Apple Slices

**Prep Time:** 10 minutes
**Cook Time:** 20 minutes
**Total Time:** 30 minutes
**Serves 4**

## INGREDIENTS

6 medium apples, sliced
2 tablespoons unsalted butter, melted
¼ cup light brown sugar
1 teaspoon ground cinnamon

Apple pie without the fattening crust. These slices make a stupendous side dish for grilled or roasted meat, a scrumptious topping for pancakes, or a delicious dessert served plain or over ice cream. Talk about versatile! When cooked, tart apples such as Granny Smiths retain their shape better than softer varieties, but may take a little longer to bake. Feel free to substitute fresh pears for the apples, or use a combination of the two.

1. Preheat oven to 450°F.

2. Place apples, butter, brown sugar, and cinnamon into a mixing bowl and toss well to coat.

3. Transfer to a shallow baking dish and cover tightly with foil. Place dish on middle rack in oven and bake for 20 minutes.

4. Remove from oven, carefully remove foil, and stir gently to recoat apples with sauce. Serve immediately.

**Per Serving (1 cup)**
Calories: 244
Fat: 6 grams
Protein: <1 gram
Sodium: 7 milligrams
Fiber: 6 grams
Carbohydrates: 51 grams
Sugar: 41 grams

# Sweet and Savory Kale with Tomatoes

**Prep Time:** 3 minutes
**Cook Time:** 12 minutes
**Total Time:** 15 minutes
**Serves 6**

## INGREDIENTS

1¼ cups low-sodium vegetable broth, divided

1 medium onion, diced

3 cloves garlic, minced

2 tablespoons salt-free prepared mustard

1 teaspoon sugar

1 tablespoon apple cider vinegar

1 pound chopped fresh kale

1 cup diced tomatoes

Freshly ground black pepper, to taste

### Kale Facts

Kale is a member of the cabbage family, grows easily in many climates, and freezes well. Once viewed as a decorative garnish, kale is increasingly taking center stage on the dinner plate. Its high levels of antioxidants make it an effective tool in the fight against cancer and cardiovascular disease. Kale contains twice the recommended daily value of vitamin A per serving, making it a valuable aid against degenerative eye diseases.

The subtle sweetness and tang in this side dish is so addictive! If garden-ripe tomatoes aren't available, substitute with salt-free canned tomatoes instead. Chop the kale into bite-sized pieces, including stems, for added fiber. Or if pressed for time, remove the thickest of the stems to speed cooking. Adapted from Rawl.net.

1. Place a large stockpot or sauté pan over medium heat. Add ¼ cup of the vegetable broth, along with the onion and garlic, and sauté for 2 minutes.

2. Add the mustard, sugar, vinegar, and remaining broth and stir to combine.

3. Add the kale and tomatoes and stir to coat. Cover the pot and cook, stirring occasionally, for 10 minutes, until kale is tender.

4. Remove from heat and season with freshly ground black pepper, to taste. Serve immediately.

**Per Serving (1 cup)**
Calories: 53
Fat: <1 gram
Protein: 2 grams
Sodium: 63 milligrams

Fiber: 2 grams
Carbohydrates: 10 grams
Sugar: 1 gram

# Lemon Parmesan Rice with Fresh Herbs

**Prep Time:** 3 minutes
**Cook Time:** 15 minutes
**Total Time:** 18 minutes
**Serves 4**

## INGREDIENTS

1 cup basmati rice

1½ cups low-sodium chicken or vegetable broth

2 tablespoons grated Parmesan cheese

2 tablespoons chopped fresh herbs

1 tablespoon freshly squeezed lemon juice

½ teaspoon grated lemon zest

½ teaspoon freshly ground black pepper

A healthy, quick, and easy low-sodium side with tons of flavor. Vary the fresh herbs to suit your mood; it's particularly tasty with parsley, cilantro, or basil. If you don't have fresh herbs on hand, substitute 1½–2 teaspoons of mixed dried herbs or your favorite all-purpose salt-free seasoning. For a cholesterol-free vegan version, choose vegetable broth and use nutritional yeast flakes instead of the cheese.

1. Rinse rice well in a fine-mesh sieve, then place in a saucepan.

2. Add broth and bring to a boil over medium-high heat. Once boiling, reduce heat to low, cover, and simmer for 15 minutes.

3. Remove pan from heat. Add remaining ingredients and stir gently to combine. Serve immediately.

**Per Serving (½ cup)**

Calories: 172
Fat: 2 grams
Protein: 6 grams
Sodium: 67 milligrams

Fiber: 1 gram
Carbohydrates: 32 grams
Sugar: 0 grams

# Braised Brussels Sprouts with Apricots and Toasted Walnuts

**Prep Time:** 5 minutes
**Cook Time:** 10 minutes
**Total Time:** 15 minutes
Serves 4

**INGREDIENTS**

¼ cup chopped walnuts

1 pound Brussels sprouts, halved

2 shallots, minced

½ cup low-sodium vegetable broth

⅓ cup diced dried apricots

¼ teaspoon freshly ground black pepper

Ready in just 15 minutes, this flavorful side is brimming with vitamins, protein, and fiber. If you don't like apricots, feel free to swap them out for dried cranberries. You can also substitute a small to medium-sized onion in place of the shallots. When cooking, add a tablespoon each of prepared salt-free mustard and agave nectar for another delicious twist on this recipe.

1. Place a sauté pan over medium heat and add walnuts. Toast, stirring, for 2 minutes. Remove from pan and set aside.

2. Return pan to heat. Add Brussels sprouts, shallots, and broth and stir to combine. Cover pan and simmer, stirring once or twice, for 8 minutes.

3. Remove from heat. Stir in apricots, the toasted walnuts, and black pepper. Serve immediately.

**Per Serving (⅔ cup)**

Calories: 120

Fat: 5 grams

Protein: 4 grams

Sodium: 43 milligrams

Fiber: 4 grams

Carbohydrates: 17 grams

Sugar: 7 grams

# Roasted Red Peppers

**Prep Time:** 5 minutes
**Cook Time:** 25 minutes
**Total Time:** 30 minutes
**Yields 1½ cups**

## INGREDIENTS

3 large red bell peppers

Roasted peppers are beautiful, tasty, and truly easy to prepare. Use them to add color, flavor, and interest to a variety of dishes, from a simple Swiss cheese and roast chicken sandwich, to a vegetarian hummus wrap, to a salad of beans, roasted onion, and corn. My favorite use? Make a tapenade with roasted pepper, low-sodium olives, nutritional yeast, dried Italian seasoning, and a tiny bit of olive oil. Pure deliciousness.

1. Preheat oven to 450°F. Take out a baking sheet and set aside.

2. Halve peppers lengthwise, then remove core and seeds.

3. Lightly spray baking sheet with oil and place peppers on the sheet, cut-side down. Place baking sheet on middle rack in oven and bake 20–25 minutes, until skins are bubbled and beginning to char.

4. Remove baking sheet from oven and place on wire rack to cool briefly. Once peppers are cool enough to handle, gently remove skins.

5. Use immediately or store in an airtight container and refrigerate until use. These also freeze well for up to 3 months if stored in a sealed, airtight container.

**Per Serving (½ cup)**

| | |
|---|---|
| Calories: 50 | Fiber: 3 grams |
| Fat: 0 grams | Carbohydrates: 9 grams |
| Protein: 1 gram | Sugar: 6 grams |
| Sodium: 6 milligrams | |

# Whipped Sweet Potatoes

Prep Time: 5 minutes
Cook Time: 20 minutes
Total Time: 25 minutes
Serves 6

## INGREDIENTS

3 medium/large sweet potatoes

3 tablespoons unsalted butter, divided

3 tablespoons brown sugar

1 tablespoon freshly squeezed orange juice

¼ teaspoon pure vanilla extract

### Whipped Butternut Squash

Puréed winter squash is a favorite rec-ipe in New England and is super easy to make. Peel a medium butternut squash, seed, then cut it into chunks. Place chunks in a microwave-safe bowl, add ¼ cup water, and cover with plastic wrap. Microwave on high for 10 minutes. Transfer contents to a food processor, add a tablespoon of low-sodium chicken or vegetable broth, and purée. Season to taste.

Perfect for holiday meals, this light and creamy sweet potato dish has hints of orange and vanilla. For more orange flavor, grate a tablespoon or two of orange zest and add to the mix. If you don't have a food processor, simply mash the sweet potatoes by hand, then whisk vigorously. The texture won't be as fluffy as if it were made in the machine, but it will come pretty close.

1. Peel sweet potatoes and cut into chunks. Place chunks in a pot and add enough water to cover by 1 or 2 inches. Place pot over high heat and bring to a boil. Once boiling, lower heat slightly, and continue cooking until tender, about 20 minutes.

2. Drain pot. Place ⅓ of the sweet potatoes into a food processor, add 1 tablespoon butter, and purée. Remove to a bowl. Repeat process with remaining sweet potatoes and butter.

3. Add the brown sugar, orange juice, and vanilla to the bowl of whipped sweet potatoes and stir well to combine. Serve immediately.

**Per Serving (⅔ cup)**
Calories: 136
Fat: 5 grams
Protein: 1 gram
Sodium: 23 grams

Fiber: 2 grams
Carbohydrates: 20 grams
Sugar: 11 grams

# Quinoa Pilaf with Mushrooms and Sage

**Prep Time:** 5 minutes
**Cook Time:** 25 minutes
**Total Time:** 30 minutes
**Serves 4**

## INGREDIENTS

2 cups low-sodium vegetable broth

1 cup quinoa, rinsed

1 tablespoon olive oil

1 medium onion, chopped

2 medium stalks celery, chopped

3 cloves garlic, minced

8 ounces mushrooms, chopped

1 teaspoon ground sage

All-purpose salt-free seasoning, to taste

Freshly ground black pepper, to taste

### Quinoa

Quinoa (pronounced KEEN-wah) was known to the ancient Incas as the mother of all grains. Its modern rise in popularity is due partly to its easy preparation. Quinoa cooks in 15 minutes and can be made successfully on the stovetop or in a rice cooker. It has a slightly nutty flavor and the individual grains have an appealing pop and chew. Quinoa is high in protein, making it a great choice for vegetarians, and because it's gluten free, it's also ideal for those with celiac disease.

This quinoa pilaf is a perfect partner for roasted lean meats, especially fowl. It's also a terrific choice for those with multiple dietary restrictions; not only is it low-sodium, but it's gluten-free and vegan, too! As such, it makes a great substitute for traditional bread dressing or stuffing at holiday meals.

1. Bring broth to a boil in a saucepan. Add quinoa. Cover pan, reduce heat to medium/low–low and simmer 20 minutes, until liquid is absorbed. Remove from heat and let sit 3–5 minutes.

2. Heat olive oil in a sauté pan over medium heat. Add onion, celery, garlic, and mushrooms and sauté until tender, about 5 minutes.

3. Add the vegetables to the quinoa. Stir in the ground sage and season to taste with salt-free seasoning and freshly ground black pepper. Serve immediately.

**Per Serving (1 cup)**

| | |
|---|---|
| Calories: 225 | Fiber: 4 grams |
| Fat: 7 grams | Carbohydrates: 32 grams |
| Protein: 10 grams | Sugar: 2 grams |
| Sodium: 58 milligrams | |

# Roasted Potatoes and Broccoli

Prep Time: 5 minutes
Cook Time: 25 minutes
Total Time: 30 minutes
Serves 6

## INGREDIENTS

4 medium potatoes, cubed

1 head fresh broccoli

1 medium onion

1 tablespoon olive oil

1 teaspoon all-purpose salt-free seasoning

½ teaspoon garlic powder

½ teaspoon ground rosemary

¼ teaspoon freshly ground black pepper

This combination of crisp, flaky potatoes and slightly smoky broccoli is so simple and so good. Peel and cube the broccoli stem and include it along with the florets; less waste, more fiber and nutrients. Change up the vegetables for variety. Add Brussels sprouts instead of broccoli, try sweet potatoes as well as regular potatoes, or use red onion for color.

1. Preheat oven to 450°F. Take out a sided baking sheet.

2. Place the cubed potatoes into a mixing bowl.

3. Cut the broccoli into florets, peel and cube the remaining stem if desired, and add to the bowl. Add the remaining ingredients and toss well to coat.

4. Spread mixture in a single layer on the baking sheet.

5. Place sheet on middle rack in oven and bake for 25 minutes. Remove from oven and serve immediately.

Per Serving (1 cup)
Calories: 153
Fat: 2 grams
Protein: 4 grams
Sodium: 48 milligrams
Fiber: 5 grams
Carbohydrates: 30 grams
Sugar: 3 grams

# Garlic Rosemary Mashed Potatoes

**Prep Time:** 10 minutes
**Cook Time:** 15 minutes
**Total Time:** 25 minutes
**Serves 6**

## INGREDIENTS

6 cups cubed red potatoes

6 cloves garlic

2 tablespoons olive oil

¼ cup low-sodium vegetable broth

1 teaspoon unflavored rice wine vinegar

1 teaspoon ground rosemary

½ teaspoon ground white pepper

¼ teaspoon dry ground mustard

Some think potatoes fall flat without the boost of salt, but these salt-free mashed potatoes, also made without butter or milk, may be the best you've ever had. White pepper adds a slightly spicier note than regular pepper and also hides well, but if you don't have any, just use standard ground black pepper. Scrub the potatoes well but keep the peels on for added nutrients and fiber.

1. Place cubed potatoes in a pot and add enough water to cover. Place pot over high heat and bring to a boil. Once boiling, reduce heat to medium-high and simmer for 15 minutes.

2. Measure remaining ingredients into a food processor and purée until smooth.

3. Remove pot from heat and drain. Mash the potatoes. Add the puréed dressing and stir well to combine.

4. Serve immediately.

**Per Serving (1 cup)**
Calories: 181
Fat: 4 grams
Protein: 3 grams
Sodium: 13 milligrams

Fiber: 3 grams
Carbohydrates: 32 grams
Sugar: 1 gram

# Carrots with Ginger, Cilantro, and Lime

**Prep Time:** 10 minutes
**Cook Time:** 11 minutes
**Total Time:** 21 minutes
**Serves 6**

## INGREDIENTS

1 tablespoon minced fresh ginger

1½ teaspoons mustard seeds

1 teaspoon freshly ground black pepper

½ teaspoon ground coriander

½ teaspoon ground cumin

¼ teaspoon salt-free curry powder

2 pounds fresh carrots

¼ cup water

1 tablespoon canola oil

Juice of 1 fresh lime

¼ cup chopped fresh cilantro

Lively and oh-so-flavorful, this carrot side is a great partner for Indian fare or grilled meat. For more spice, add half of a minced jalapeño pepper along with the other seasonings. When buying commercial curry powder, be sure to check the ingredients list carefully; many brands contain hidden salt. Adapted from *Hannaford Fresh* magazine.

1. Measure the ginger, mustard seeds, black pepper, coriander, cumin, and curry powder into a small bowl. Mix and set aside.

2. Peel the carrots and cut diagonally into roughly ½-inch slices.

3. Place a sauté pan over medium heat. Add the water, oil, and carrots to the pan and bring to a boil. Cover pan and cook, shaking occasionally, until carrots are just barely tender, about 7 minutes.

4. Uncover the pan and continue to cook until carrots begin to sizzle in the oil, about 2 minutes.

5. Add the spice mixture and cook, stirring constantly, for 2 minutes. Remove from heat.

6. Add the lime juice and cilantro and stir to combine. Serve immediately.

**Per Serving (1 cup)**
Calories: 74
Fat: 2 grams
Protein: 1 gram
Sodium: 117 milligrams

Fiber: 4 grams
Carbohydrates: 12 grams
Sugar: 7 grams

# Southwestern Rice Pilaf

**Prep Time:** 5 minutes
**Cook Time:** 25 minutes
**Total Time:** 30 minutes
**Serves 4**

## INGREDIENTS

1 tablespoon olive oil

1 medium red onion, diced

4 cloves garlic, minced

1 medium red bell pepper, diced

1 small green bell pepper, diced

2 teaspoons salt-free chili seasoning

1 teaspoon ground cumin

1½ cups long-grain rice

2½ cups low-sodium vegetable broth

1 (15-ounce) can no-salt-added diced tomatoes

1 jalapeño pepper, minced

¼ cup chopped fresh cilantro

Filling and flavorful, this easy rice pilaf partners perfectly with Tex-Mex dishes, burgers, and refried beans. If you're not a fan of spice, feel free to omit the jalapeño pepper altogether, or simply remove the seeds before mincing to curtail its kick. Salt-free canned tomatoes are sold readily at supermarkets; feel free to substitute an equal amount of chopped fresh tomatoes during the summer season. Adapted from *Fine Cooking*.

1. Heat olive oil in a large lidded saucepan over medium heat. Add the onion, garlic, and bell peppers and sauté for 2 minutes.

2. Add the chili seasoning and cumin and sauté for 3 minutes.

3. Add the rice and stir well to coat. Reduce heat to medium-low and cook, stirring, for 2 minutes.

4. Add the broth and tomatoes and stir well. Raise heat to high and bring to a boil. Once boiling, reduce heat to low, cover securely, and simmer for 18 minutes. Remove from heat and let sit for 5 minutes.

5. Remove lid, add the jalapeño and cilantro, and gently fold in. Serve immediately.

**Per Serving (1¾ cups)**

Calories: 304

Fat: 4 grams

Protein: 7 grams

Sodium: 105 milligrams

Fiber: 4 grams

Carbohydrates: 57 grams

Sugar: 5 grams

# Curried Butternut Squash

**Prep Time:** 5 minutes
**Cook Time:** 25 minutes
**Total Time:** 30 minutes
**Serves 4**

## INGREDIENTS

1 medium butternut squash (about 2½ cups cubed)

2 tablespoons unsalted butter

1 teaspoon salt-free curry powder

Butternut squash is so healthy and, thanks to modern-day convenience, can even be purchased pre-peeled and cubed. This is a delicious dish to turn to for both casual meals and holiday affairs. The roasting process brings out the sweetness of the squash, and the curry adds a savory dimension that's truly out of this world. Adapted from *Taste of Home: Dinner on a Dime*.

1. Preheat oven to 450°F. Take out a 9" × 13" baking dish and set aside.

2. Place squash on a cutting board. Trim off the top and bottom, then carefully peel. Slice in half and remove seeds using a spoon. Cut into 1-inch cubes and set aside.

3. Place butter in baking dish and put dish into oven. Watch, and remove as soon as the butter has melted. Sprinkle curry powder over the melted butter, then add the cubed squash, and toss until evenly coated.

4. Place baking dish on middle rack in oven and roast 20–25 minutes, until squash is tender and very lightly browned. Remove from oven and serve immediately.

**Per Serving (⅔ cup)**
Calories: 113
Fat: 6 grams
Protein: 2 grams
Sodium: 8 milligrams
Fiber: 2 grams
Carbohydrates: 17 grams
Sugar: 3 grams

# Sautéed Spinach with Onions and Garlic

**Prep Time:** 3 minutes
**Cook Time:** 7 minutes
**Total Time:** 10 minutes
**Serves 2**

## INGREDIENTS

1 teaspoon olive oil

1 small onion, minced

2 cloves garlic, minced

6 cups fresh spinach, washed well

Freshly ground black pepper, to taste

A deliciously healthy side in just 10 minutes. Baby spinach requires nothing more than a good rinsing. When using larger spinach leaves, wash well, remove tough stems, then chop. For variety, add 8 ounces of sliced mushrooms during cooking. The earthy taste and toothsome texture marries perfectly with the mix. Or substitute other dark leafy greens, such as Swiss chard or kale, adjusting cooking time accordingly.

1. Heat olive oil in a sauté pan over medium heat. Add the onion and garlic and sauté for 2 minutes.

2. Add the spinach and sauté just until wilted, roughly 3–5 minutes. Remove from heat.

3. Season with freshly ground black pepper, to taste. Serve immediately.

**Per Serving (1 cup)**

| | |
|---|---|
| Calories: 52 | Fiber: 2 grams |
| Fat: 2 grams | Carbohydrates: 6 grams |
| Protein: 3 grams | Sugar: 0 grams |
| Sodium: 72 milligrams | |

# Stir-Fried Cabbage and Noodles

**Prep Time:** 5 minutes
**Cook Time:** 10 minutes
**Total Time:** 15 minutes
Serves 6

## INGREDIENTS

8 ounces yolkless wide egg noodles

1 tablespoon olive oil

½ medium head green cabbage, chopped

1 medium onion, chopped

1 teaspoon caraway seeds

All-purpose salt-free seasoning, to taste

Freshly ground black pepper, to taste

This is the type of dish you could live off of all winter. Hearty, healthy, cheap, and filling. It's a great change from standard stuffing or potato sides, and makes a great one-dish meal when combined with cooked chicken or turkey. The combination of flavors is fantastic, especially the little rush you get each time you bite open one of the tiny caraway seeds. Adapted from the American Heart Association's *Low-Salt Cookbook*.

1. Prepare noodles according to package directions, omitting salt. Drain and set aside.

2. Heat olive oil in a large sauté pan over medium heat. Add cabbage and onion and sauté for 5–8 minutes, until tender crisp.

3. Stir in prepared noodles, caraway seeds, salt-free seasoning and freshly ground black pepper, to taste.

4. Serve immediately.

**Per Serving (1 cup)**
Calories: 138
Fat: 3 grams
Protein: 4 grams
Sodium: 22 milligrams
Fiber: 3 grams
Carbohydrates: 23 grams
Sugar: 3 grams

# Rice with Black Beans, Mango, and Lime

**Prep Time:** 10 minutes
**Cook Time:** 0 minutes
**Total Time:** 10 minutes
Serves 6

## INGREDIENTS

3 cups cooked rice

1 (15-ounce) can no-salt-added black beans, drained

1 ripe mango, diced

1 medium red bell pepper, diced

2 scallions, sliced

2 cloves garlic, minced

Juice of 2 fresh limes

¼ cup chopped fresh cilantro

Freshly ground black pepper, to taste

This low-fat, virtually sodium-free side is a fabulous way to re-use leftover rice. Delicious warm or cold, it showcases simple, fresh flavors the best way possible: naked! Use whatever cooked rice you have on hand: brown, basmati, jasmine, and even wild rice all work well. If you don't have mango, substitute an equal amount of diced pineapple.

1. Place all the ingredients into a mixing bowl and stir well to combine.

2. Serve immediately or cover and refrigerate until ready to serve.

**Per Serving (1 cup)**

| | |
|---|---|
| Calories: 230 | Fiber: 7 grams |
| Fat: 1 gram | Carbohydrates: 47 grams |
| Protein: 9 grams | Sugar: 6 grams |
| Sodium: 4 milligrams | |

# Sun-Dried Tomato Couscous with Pine Nuts and Basil

**Prep Time:** 15 minutes
**Cook Time:** 10 minutes
**Total Time:** 25 minutes
Serves 4

## INGREDIENTS

1 cup chopped sun-dried tomatoes

2 cups boiling water

1 cup dry whole-grain couscous

2 teaspoons olive oil

4 cloves garlic, minced

⅓ cup pine nuts

¼ teaspoon freshly ground black pepper

2 tablespoons chopped fresh basil

Sun-dried tomatoes do double duty in this flavorful whole-grain couscous, providing an astronomical amount of flavor with absolutely no salt. Select sun-dried tomatoes stored without oil. If you don't have sun-dried tomatoes, substitute 2 cups low-sodium tomato or vegetable juice for the water and add a 15-ounce can of salt-free diced tomatoes instead.

1. Place the sun-dried tomatoes in a small bowl and add the boiling water. Let sit for 15 minutes.

2. Pour off the soaking liquid into a measuring cup and add enough water to make 2 cups. Set tomatoes aside.

3. Pour the liquid into a saucepan and bring to a boil over high heat. Once boiling, stir in the couscous, reduce heat to medium-low, cover, and simmer for 2 minutes.

4. Remove pot from heat, remove lid, and fluff couscous with a fork. Set aside to cool for 5 minutes.

5. Heat olive oil in a sauté pan over medium heat. Add the tomatoes, garlic, and pine nuts and sauté for 3 minutes. Remove from heat.

6. Add couscous, pepper, and basil and toss well to combine. Serve immediately.

**Per Serving (¾ cup)**
Calories: 275
Fat: 11 grams
Protein: 8 grams
Sodium: 282 milligrams

Fiber: 4 grams
Carbohydrates: 37 grams
Sugar: 6 grams

# Garlic Steamed Squash

**Prep Time:** 5 minutes
**Cook Time:** 10 minutes
**Total Time:** 15 minutes
**Serves 4**

## INGREDIENTS

2 small/medium yellow squash

2 small/medium zucchini

6 cloves garlic, peeled

All-purpose salt-free seasoning, to taste

Freshly ground black pepper, to taste

One of the simplest sides ever: fat-free, almost sodium-free, yet so much flavor! Slice yellow squash and zucchini, toss them into a steamer with some garlic cloves, and in 10 minutes it's ready. When steamed, the garlic softens like magic, making it oh-so mellow and irresistible. Serious garlic fans may want to pop in a whole peeled head.

1. Trim the squash and zucchini and cut into 1-inch rounds.

2. Fill a steamer pot about 1 inch deep with water. Place pot over high heat and bring to a boil.

3. Place the veggies and garlic into the steamer basket. Place the steamer basket into the pot and cover tightly with lid. Steam for 10 minutes.

4. Remove pot from heat and carefully remove lid. Pluck garlic cloves from pot and gently mash with a fork.

5. Transfer the steamed veggies to a serving bowl, add the mashed garlic and toss gently to coat. Season to taste with all-purpose salt-free seasoning and freshly ground black pepper. Serve immediately.

**Per Serving (1 cup)**

| | |
|---|---|
| Calories: 38 | Fiber: 2 grams |
| Fat: 0 grams | Carbohydrates: 8 grams |
| Protein: 2 grams | Sugar: 4 grams |
| Sodium: 5 milligrams | |

# CHAPTER 7

# Main Meat Dishes

Broccoli, Ground Turkey, and Pesto Pizza

Basil Pesto

Lemon Thyme Turkey Meatballs

Ground Turkey Meatloaf Minis

Sesame Chicken with Couscous

Faux Soy Sauce

Spicy Sweet-and-Sour Chicken

Low-Sodium Kung Pao Chicken

Chicken, Black Bean, and Veggie Soft Tacos

Salt-Free Chili Seasoning

Grilled Tequila Chicken with Sautéed Peppers and Onion

Oven-Baked Chicken Tenders

Stovetop Barbecued Chicken Bites

Spicy, Sweet, and Tangy Barbecue Sauce

Chicken Curry with Creamy Tomato Sauce

Easy Spaghetti and Meatballs

30-Minute Ground Beef Pizza

Beef Tacos

Cajun-Style Dirty Rice

Quick and Easy Shepherd's Pie

Lamb Chops with Rosemary

Ginger and Garlic Pork Stir-Fry

Asian-Inspired Mini Meatloaves with Salt-Free Hoisin Glaze

Barbecue Pizza with Ground Pork, Peppers, and Pineapple

Southwestern Salmon

Baked Tuna Cakes

Pasta with Cherry Tomatoes, Tuna, and Lemon

Tuna Noodle Casserole

Healthy Fish and Chips

Shrimp Creole

# Broccoli, Ground Turkey, and Pesto Pizza

**Prep Time:** 5 minutes
**Cook Time:** 25 minutes
**Total Time:** 30 minutes
**Serves 4**

## INGREDIENTS

1 cup white whole-wheat flour

1 teaspoon all-purpose salt-free seasoning

1 teaspoon salt-free Italian seasoning

½ teaspoon garlic powder

2 egg whites

⅔ cup low-fat milk

½ pound lean ground turkey

1 medium red onion, chopped

1 medium red bell pepper, diced

1 teaspoon olive oil

1 head broccoli, chopped

4 tablespoons Basil Pesto (see recipe in this chapter)

½ cup Swiss cheese, shredded

Freshly ground black pepper, to taste

Tasty ground turkey, savory red onion, broccoli, and pesto make this a low-sodium pizza you won't forget. And the very best part? It's table-ready in just 30 minutes! Substitute lean ground chicken if you prefer. If you don't have time to make pesto, spoon commercial salt-free pasta sauce over the baked crust instead; sprinkle liberally with salt-free seasoning and dried Italian herbs like basil, oregano, and thyme.

1. Preheat oven to 450°F. Grease and flour a 12-inch nonstick pizza pan and set aside.

2. Measure the flour, seasonings, and garlic powder into a mixing bowl and whisk well to combine. Add the egg whites and milk and stir well. Pour batter into the prepared pizza pan, spread batter to edges, and set aside.

3. Place a large skillet over medium heat. Add the ground turkey, onion, and bell pepper and cook, stirring, for 5 minutes.

4. Remove from heat and carefully drain any excess fat. Spoon mixture evenly over the batter in the pan. Place pan on middle rack in oven and bake for 15 minutes.

5. While pizza is baking, heat olive oil in a sauté pan over medium heat. Add the broccoli and sauté for 5 minutes. Remove pan from heat and set aside.

6. Remove pan from oven and top pizza with pesto, spreading evenly. Arrange broccoli evenly over top, then sprinkle with Swiss cheese and freshly ground black pepper, to taste. Return pan to oven

continued on next page

and bake for 5 minutes, until cheese has melted completely.

7. Remove pizza from oven. Gently remove from pan and cut into 8 slices. Serve immediately.

**Per Serving (2 slices)**

| | |
|---|---|
| Calories: 327 | Fiber: 5 grams |
| Fat: 14 grams | Carbohydrates: 30 grams |
| Protein: 22 grams | Sugar: 4 grams |
| Sodium: 131 milligrams | |

# Basil Pesto

**Prep Time:** 3 minutes
**Cook Time:** 0 minutes
**Total Time:** 3 minutes
**Yields ½ cup**

## INGREDIENTS

2 cups fresh basil leaves

4 cloves garlic

3 tablespoons olive oil

¼ cup walnuts, almonds, or pine nuts

2 tablespoons grated Parmesan cheese

¼ teaspoon freshly ground black pepper

Harvest that fragrant bounty of basil and enjoy it to its fullest. Stir a little bit into pasta or rice for a taste sensation, or use it as a spread for sandwiches, a topping for pizza, and more. For an equally delicious cholesterol-free (vegan) version, substitute 2–3 tablespoons of nutritional yeast flakes for the Parmesan cheese.

1. Place all the ingredients into a food processor and pulse until smooth.

2. Use immediately or store in an airtight container and refrigerate until use.

**Per Serving (2 tablespoons)**

Calories: 166

Fat: 17 grams

Protein: 2 grams

Sodium: 39 milligrams

Fiber: <1 gram

Carbohydrates: 2 grams

Sugar: <1 gram

# Lemon Thyme Turkey Meatballs

**Prep Time:** 7 minutes
**Cook Time:** 23 minutes
**Total Time:** 30 minutes
Serves 6

## INGREDIENTS

¼ cup white whole-wheat flour

1 medium onion, cut into chunks

3 cloves garlic

Grated zest of 1 fresh lemon

1½ teaspoons dried thyme, divided

1 pound lean ground turkey

¾ cup salt-free bread crumbs

3 tablespoons grated Parmesan cheese

¼ teaspoon freshly ground black pepper

2 teaspoons olive oil

½ cup dry white wine

1¾ cups low-sodium chicken broth

1½ tablespoons freshly squeezed lemon juice

Juicy inside with a crunchy outer crust, each bite of these meatballs is infused with a hint of citrus and the heavenly scent of thyme. The light and creamy sauce incorporates the same tastes and aromas, bringing this salt-free dish to unparalleled heights of flavor. Serve over whole-grain noodles, cooked rice, or quinoa. Adapted from *EatingWell* magazine.

1. Place flour into a shallow bowl and set aside.

2. Place onion, garlic, and lemon zest in a food processor. Add 1 teaspoon dried thyme and pulse briefly to combine.

3. Transfer mixture to a large bowl and add in the turkey, bread crumbs, Parmesan, and pepper. Mix, using your hands, until combined. Pinch off 2 tablespoons at a time and shape into meatballs.

4. Roll the meatballs in the flour to lightly coat. Reserve the remaining flour.

5. Heat the olive oil in a sauté pan over medium heat. Add the coated meatballs and cook, turning once or twice, until browned, about 5 minutes. Remove the meatballs from the pan and set aside.

6. Add wine to the pan, increase heat to medium-high, and cook, scraping up any browned bits, until almost evaporated, about 1 minute.

7. Add the broth and bring to a boil. Reduce heat to maintain a simmer and return the meatballs to the pan along with the remaining thyme. Cover and cook until the meatballs are cooked through, about 10 minutes.

continued on next page

8. Remove the meatballs again and set aside. Bring the sauce to a boil over medium-high heat and cook until reduced to about 1 cup, roughly 5 minutes.

9. Add the lemon juice and 1 tablespoon of the flour into a small bowl and whisk until smooth. Add this flour mixture to the sauce and simmer, whisking constantly, until slightly thickened, roughly 1–2 minutes.

10. Remove the pan from heat and add meatballs, swirling to coat. Serve immediately, seasoned with freshly ground black pepper, to taste.

**Per Serving (⅙ of the meatballs)**

| | |
|---|---|
| Calories: 226 | Fiber: 1 gram |
| Fat: 8 grams | Carbohydrates: 17 grams |
| Protein: 20 grams | Sugar: 1 gram |
| Sodium: 117 milligrams | |

# Ground Turkey Meatloaf Minis

Prep Time: 5 minutes
Cook Time: 25 minutes
Total Time: 30 minutes
Serves 6

## INGREDIENTS

1½ pounds lean ground turkey

1 medium onion, finely diced

2 medium stalks celery, finely diced

1 small bell pepper, finely diced

4 cloves garlic, minced

1 (8-ounce) can no-salt-added tomato sauce

1 egg white

¾ cup salt-free bread crumbs

1 tablespoon molasses

¼ teaspoon liquid smoke

½ teaspoon dried basil

½ teaspoon dried oregano

½ teaspoon dried savory

½ teaspoon dried thyme

½ teaspoon freshly ground black pepper

¼ cup salt-free ketchup

### Homemade Bread Crumbs

To make your own salt-free bread crumbs, crisp several pieces of salt-free or low-sodium bread in the toaster or conventional oven. Tear or crumb the toasted bread into tiny pieces. For a finer crumb, pulse the bread pieces in a food processor. Wonderful low-sodium bread crumb substitutes can also be made from finely chopped unsalted nuts, matzo, and salt-free potato chips.

A deliciously lighter version of the all-American meal, these mini meatloaves can also be made with lean ground chicken. Serve with Garlic Rosemary Mashed Potatoes (see recipe in Chapter 6: Appetizers and Side Dishes) and fresh green beans sautéed with garlic. If you don't have salt-free bread crumbs, substitute an equal amount of quick oats instead.

1. Preheat oven to 400°F. Spray a 6-cup jumbo muffin tin lightly with oil and set aside.

2. Place all of the ingredients except ketchup into a large bowl and mix well using your hands.

3. Divide mixture evenly between the muffin cups and press in firmly.

4. Divide the ketchup between the muffin cups and spread evenly for a nice glaze.

5. Place muffin tin on middle rack in oven and bake for 25 minutes.

6. Remove from oven. Gently run a knife around each loaf and remove from tin. Serve immediately.

**Per Serving (1 mini meatloaf)**

| | |
|---|---|
| Calories: 251 | Fiber: 2 grams |
| Fat: 7 grams | Carbohydrates: 21 grams |
| Protein: 25 grams | Sugar: 7 grams |
| Sodium: 112 milligrams | |

# Sesame Chicken with Couscous

**Prep Time:** 10 minutes
**Cook Time:** 8 minutes
**Total Time:** 18 minutes
**Serves 4**

## INGREDIENTS

1½ cups low-sodium chicken broth

3 teaspoons Faux Soy Sauce, divided (see recipe in this chapter)

2 teaspoons sesame oil, divided

1 cup uncooked couscous

2 scallions, sliced (green and white portions)

1 large red bell pepper, diced

1½ cups snow peas or sugar snap peas

1 cup broccoli florets

1 cup cooked chicken, cubed

3 tablespoons lemon juice

2 tablespoons olive oil

Freshly ground black pepper, to taste

1 tablespoon toasted sesame seeds

This low-sodium reinvention of a classic Chinese favorite is simply irresistible; one bite and you'll be hooked! The sweet, tangy chicken is still there, but the fried batter is replaced with fluffy and flavorful couscous. Add in tender-crisp veggies, a savory lemon-sesame dressing, and toasted sesame seeds, and it's a dish you'll devour. Substitute commercial low-sodium soy sauce for the Faux Soy Sauce, if desired. Adapted from *Simply in Season.*

1. Measure the chicken broth, 1 teaspoon faux soy sauce, and 1 teaspoon sesame oil into a saucepan. Bring to a boil over high heat. Once boiling, remove from heat, add couscous, stir, and cover. Let stand 5 minutes.

2. Transfer cooked couscous to a bowl. Add the sliced scallion and diced bell pepper and stir well to combine. Set aside.

3. Take out a stockpot with steamer insert. Place 2 inches water in the stockpot and bring to a boil over high heat. Put the peas into the steamer basket, and once water is boiling, place basket into the stockpot. Cover and steam 1 minute. Remove lid and add broccoli to the basket; replace lid and steam 2 minutes more. Remove from heat. Rinse peas and broccoli under cold water and drain. Add the peas and broccoli to the couscous mixture, along with the cubed cooked chicken.

4. Measure the lemon juice, olive oil, 2 teaspoons faux soy sauce, 1 teaspoon sesame oil, and freshly

continued on next page

ground black pepper into a small mixing bowl and whisk well to combine. Pour over the couscous mixture, add the toasted sesame seeds, and toss well to combine.

5. Serve immediately.

**Per Serving (1½ cups)**

| | |
|---|---|
| Calories: 378 | Fiber: 5 grams |
| Fat: 12 grams | Carbohydrates: 49 grams |
| Protein: 19 grams | Sugar: 8 grams |
| Sodium: 70 milligrams | |

# Faux Soy Sauce

**Prep Time:** 2 minutes
**Cook Time:** 1 minute
**Total Time:** 3 minutes
**Yields** ⅔ cup

## INGREDIENTS

¼ cup molasses

3 tablespoons unflavored rice wine vinegar

1 tablespoon water

1 teaspoon sodium-free beef bouillon granules

½ teaspoon freshly ground black pepper

### Molasses Alert!

When making Faux Soy Sauce and other dishes, look for the lowest-sodium molasses you can find. Grandma's Original Molasses (unsulphured) and Crosby's Fancy Molasses are both very low in sodium. If you can't locate either, check labels carefully before purchase. Some molasses brands contain high levels of sodium; it's better to be safe than sorry.

Meet soy sauce's tasty cousin, Faux. If you've never used this Faux concoction before, just wait till you *taste* its marvelous effect! On its own it won't pass for soy sauce, though it shares the same deep dark look. But once added into a recipe it melds with the other flavors to produce the most remarkable fake-out ever. Sodium-free beef bouillon granules are located alongside traditional high-sodium bouillon cubes in the soup aisle of most supermarkets. Adapted from Dick Logue's Soy Sauce Substitute in *500 Low Sodium Recipes*.

1. Measure all the ingredients into a small saucepan or microwave-safe bowl and heat on low to combine, roughly 1 minute.

2. Use immediately or store in an airtight container and refrigerate until ready to use.

**Per Serving (1 tablespoon)**
Calories: 25
Fat: 0 grams
Protein: 0 grams
Sodium: 3 milligrams
Fiber: 0 grams
Carbohydrates: 6 grams
Sugar: 4 grams

# Spicy Sweet-and-Sour Chicken

**Prep Time:** 10 minutes
**Cook Time:** 8 minutes
**Total Time:** 18 minutes
**Serves 4**

## INGREDIENTS

1 pound boneless, skinless chicken breasts, cut into 1-inch cubes

2 tablespoons cornstarch, divided

3 tablespoons Faux Soy Sauce, divided (see recipe in this chapter)

1 (8-ounce) can pineapple chunks, in juice (liquid reserved)

¼ cup apple cider vinegar

¼ cup sugar

2 tablespoons salt-free ketchup

2 teaspoons sriracha

½ teaspoon ground ginger

1 tablespoon vegetable oil

1 small onion, diced

2 cloves garlic, minced

1 medium bell pepper, diced

If you adore Asian cooking, here's another must-try recipe. Spicy, sweet, and tangy bites of tender chicken simmered with pineapple, onion, and green pepper in a flavorful low-sodium sauce. Sriracha is a bottled red chili sauce sold in the "international foods" section of many supermarkets. If you can't find it, substitute an equal amount of hot sauce or dried red pepper flakes to taste. Adapted from *Cooking Light* magazine.

1. Wash chicken breasts and pat dry. Combine chicken, 1 tablespoon cornstarch, and 1 tablespoon faux soy sauce in a small bowl; toss well to coat. Set aside.

2. Drain liquid from the pineapple into another small bowl. Then measure in the remaining tablespoon cornstarch, remaining 2 tablespoons faux soy sauce, vinegar, sugar, salt-free ketchup, sriracha, and ginger; whisk to combine. Set aside.

3. Heat a large skillet over medium-high heat. Add the vegetable oil and swirl to coat. Add chicken to pan and cook, stirring, 3 minutes. Add onion and garlic and sauté 1 minute. Stir in pineapple and bell pepper and cook, stirring, 3 minutes. Stir in the sauce mixture and cook, stirring constantly, 1 minute.

4. Remove from heat and serve immediately.

**Per Serving (1½ cups)**
Calories: 292
Fat: 5 grams
Protein: 27 grams
Sodium: 143 milligrams

Fiber: 1 gram
Carbohydrates: 33 grams
Sugar: 26 grams

# Low-Sodium Kung Pao Chicken

**Prep Time:** 10 minutes
**Cook Time:** 10 minutes
**Total Time:** 20 minutes
**Serves 4**

## INGREDIENTS

1 cup low-sodium chicken broth

2 tablespoons Faux Soy Sauce (see recipe in this chapter)

1 tablespoon balsamic vinegar

5 tablespoons cornstarch, divided

2 teaspoons sesame oil

1 teaspoon sugar

1 pound boneless, skinless chicken breasts, cubed

¼ teaspoon freshly ground black pepper

2 tablespoons canola oil, divided

¼ teaspoon dried red pepper flakes

2 tablespoons minced fresh ginger

6 scallions, sliced, whites and greens kept separate

1 medium red bell pepper, cubed

2 medium stalks celery, sliced

2 medium carrots, sliced

¼ cup plain unflavored rice vinegar

¼ cup unsalted cashews or peanuts, chopped

The spicy bite of ginger, the tang of rice wine vinegar, the smoky depth of sesame oil, that certain indescribable something that says "I am Chinese takeout"—it's all here! With careful adaptation (in this case, using Faux Soy Sauce instead of regular), you can achieve a fantastic level of flavor with a fraction of the sodium. Adapted from *Fine Cooking*.

1. Place the chicken broth, faux soy sauce, balsamic vinegar, 1 tablespoon cornstarch, sesame oil, and sugar into a bowl. Whisk well to combine and set aside.

2. Place the chicken into a mixing bowl, add 4 tablespoons cornstarch and black pepper and toss well to coat using a pair of tongs.

3. Heat 1 tablespoon canola oil in a sauté pan over medium heat. Add the chicken and cook until lightly browned on all sides, about 4 minutes total.

4. Add the remaining tablespoon oil to the pan. Add the red pepper flakes, ginger, and whites of the scallions and cook, stirring, for 1 minute.

5. Add the bell pepper, celery, and carrots and sauté until they soften slightly, about 2 minutes.

6. Add the rice vinegar and scrape the bottom of the pan to incorporate any browned bits. Give the chicken broth mixture a quick whisk, then add to the pan.

7. Check the chicken. If still pink inside, reduce heat and cook a couple minutes more. Remove pan from heat and serve immediately, sprinkled with the chopped nuts and scallion greens.

**Per Serving (1½ cups)**

| | |
|---|---|
| Calories: 347 | Fiber: 2 grams |
| Fat: 14 grams | Carbohydrates: 24 grams |
| Protein: 29 grams | Sugar: 8 grams |
| Sodium: 135 milligrams | |

# Chicken, Black Bean, and Veggie Soft Tacos

**Prep Time:** 10 minutes
**Cook Time:** 15 minutes
**Total Time:** 25 minutes
**Serves 6**

## INGREDIENTS

1 package 5-inch corn tortillas

3 boneless, skinless chicken thighs

½ cup low-sodium chicken broth

1 medium carrot, diced

1 medium sweet potato, diced

1 medium onion, diced

1 medium bell pepper, diced

1 jalapeño pepper, minced

3 cloves garlic, minced

1 (15-ounce) can no-salt-added black beans

½ cup corn kernels

2 tablespoons no-salt-added tomato paste

2 tablespoons Salt-Free Chili Seasoning (see recipe in this chapter)

½ cup nonfat sour cream

¼ cup chopped fresh cilantro

Soft corn tortillas filled with a spicy combination of chicken, veggies, and beans. A recipe for homemade Salt-Free Chili Seasoning is provided in this chapter. If you're using a commercial chili seasoning instead, be sure to start with just a teaspoon and work up from there. Some brands can be quite fiery and you don't want to risk over-seasoning.

1. Warm corn tortillas as desired. Set aside.

2. Wash the chicken and cut into bite-sized pieces. Set aside.

3. Heat a sauté pan over medium heat. Add the broth, carrot, and sweet potato, cover the pan, and cook for 5 minutes.

4. Add the chicken, onion, peppers, and garlic. Cover, and cook for another 5 minutes, stirring once halfway through cooking time.

5. Add the beans (including liquid), corn, tomato paste, and chili seasoning to the pan. Stir well and cook, continuing to stir, for 5 minutes.

6. Remove from heat. Spoon filling into warm tortillas and garnish with sour cream and cilantro.

7. Serve immediately.

**Per Serving (2 tacos)**

| | |
|---|---|
| Calories: 338 | Fiber: 9 grams |
| Fat: 3 grams | Carbohydrates: 63 grams |
| Protein: 17 grams | Sugar: 5 grams |
| Sodium: 90 milligrams | |

# Salt-Free Chili Seasoning

**Prep Time:** 5 minutes
**Cook Time:** 0 minutes
**Total Time:** 5 minutes
**Yields ⅔ cup (5 servings)**

## INGREDIENTS

2 tablespoons ground cumin

1 tablespoon ground coriander

2 teaspoons dried oregano

1½ teaspoons ground sweet paprika

½ teaspoon dried red pepper flakes

½ teaspoon garlic powder

½ teaspoon onion powder

¼ teaspoon dry ground mustard

⅛ teaspoon ground cayenne pepper

If you have difficulty finding commercial salt-free chili seasoning, make your own! It's quick, affordable, and best yet, the individual seasonings can be adjusted to suit your taste. After assembling the seasoning, store in a tightly sealed container in a cool, dark place. Although it's convenient to keep spices on the counter, it compromises their flavor.

1. Measure all the ingredients into a small mixing bowl and whisk well to combine.

2. Store seasoning in a small lidded jar.

**Per Serving (1 tablespoon)**

Calories: 0
Fat: 0 grams
Protein: 0 grams
Sodium: 0 grams

Fiber: 0 grams
Carbohydrates: 0 grams
Sugar: 0 grams

# Grilled Tequila Chicken with Sautéed Peppers and Onion

**Prep Time:** 5 minutes
**Cook Time:** 25 minutes
**Total Time:** 30 minutes
**Serves 4**

## INGREDIENTS

1 cup lime juice

⅓ cup tequila

3 cloves garlic, chopped

¼ cup chopped fresh cilantro

1 tablespoon agave nectar

½ teaspoon freshly ground black pepper

1 teaspoon cumin

½ teaspoon ground coriander

4 boneless, skinless chicken breasts

2 teaspoons canola oil

1 large green bell pepper, diced

1 large red bell pepper, diced

1 large onion, diced

½ cup nonfat sour cream

Thanks to the tequila marinade, this fabulous chicken dish is succulent, moist, and unbelievably flavorful. The longer the chicken steeps, the greater the flavor, so if possible, make the marinade first thing in the morning and let the chicken steep all day. Serve with fresh corn on the cob, nonfat sour cream, and chopped fresh cilantro.

1. Measure the lime juice, tequila, garlic, cilantro, agave nectar, black pepper, cumin, and coriander into a mixing bowl and whisk well to combine.

2. Wash chicken breasts and pat dry. Add to mixture and turn several times to coat. Cover and refrigerate. Allow to marinate for at least 6 hours, preferably overnight.

3. Heat the grill. Once ready, cook chicken until no longer pink but still juicy and tender, about 10 minutes per side.

4. While chicken is grilling, heat the oil in a sauté pan over medium heat. Add the diced peppers and onion and cook, stirring, for 5 minutes. Remove from heat.

5. Remove chicken from grill. Plate each breast with ¼ of the veggies and a dollop of sour cream. Serve immediately.

**Per Serving (1 chicken breast)**
Calories: 259
Fat: 3 grams
Protein: 28 grams
Sodium: 118 milligrams

Fiber: 1 gram
Carbohydrates: 18 grams
Sugar: 7 grams

# Oven-Baked Chicken Tenders

**Prep Time:** 10 minutes
**Cook Time:** 15 minutes
**Total Time:** 25 minutes
**Serves 8**

## INGREDIENTS

3 pounds boneless, skinless chicken breast tenderloins

½ cup unbleached all-purpose flour

½ cup white whole-wheat flour

½ cup salt-free bread crumbs

2 teaspoons garlic powder

2 teaspoons onion powder

1 teaspoon ground sweet paprika

1 teaspoon freshly ground black pepper

½ cup low-fat milk

1 egg white

This remarkable recipe yields restaurant-style chicken tenders that are as healthy as they are delicious! Baked rather than fried, these crispy tenders are much lower in fat, but still full of flavor. As a bonus, they freeze wonderfully. Double or triple the recipe and freeze left-overs for later meals. Serve with salt-free ketchup, BBQ sauce, or honey for dipping.

1. Preheat oven to 375°F. Take out a large baking sheet, cover with aluminum foil, spray lightly with oil, and set aside.

2. Wash the chicken and pat dry.

3. Combine the flours, bread crumbs, and seasonings in a large zip-top plastic bag. Seal and shake well to combine.

4. In a shallow bowl, whisk together the milk and egg white.

5. One piece at a time, dip the chicken into the milk mixture, then place in the flour bag, seal, and shake vigorously to coat. Place breaded tenders on the prepared baking sheet.

6. Place baking sheet on middle rack in oven and bake for 10–15 minutes, until golden brown, turning once halfway through cooking time.

7. Remove from oven and serve immediately.

**Per Serving (⅛ of the chicken tenders)**

| | |
|---|---|
| Calories: 266 | Fiber: 1 gram |
| Fat: 2 grams | Carbohydrates: 13 grams |
| Protein: 45 grams | Sugar: 1 gram |
| Sodium: 132 milligrams | |

# Stovetop Barbecued Chicken Bites

**Prep Time:** 10 minutes
**Cook Time:** 20 minutes
**Total Time:** 30 minutes
**Serves 4**

## INGREDIENTS

1 pound boneless skinless chicken breasts

1 tablespoon canola oil

1 medium onion, diced

3 cloves garlic, minced

1 medium bell pepper, diced

1 cup Spicy, Sweet, and Tangy Barbecue Sauce (see recipe in this chapter)

Freshly ground black pepper, to taste

Forget standing outside over a grill! Here's a recipe for delicious barbecued chicken you can whip up anytime! Succulent bites of tender chicken are simmered with onion, garlic, and bell pepper in a tangy low-sodium barbecue sauce. Serve over baked potatoes, cooked rice, or quinoa. Or for a tasty meal, partner with Sweet Corn Muffins (see recipe in Chapter 2: Breakfasts) and Creamy Low-Sodium Coleslaw (recipe in Chapter 3: Salads and Dressings).

1. Wash chicken breasts and pat dry. Cut into bite-sized chunks.

2. Heat oil in a large sauté pan over medium heat. Add chicken, onion, garlic, and bell pepper, and cook, stirring, for 5 minutes.

3. Add the barbecue sauce and stir to combine. Reduce heat to medium-low and cover pan. Cook, stirring frequently, until chicken is fully cooked, about 15 minutes.

4. Remove from heat. Season to taste with freshly ground black pepper and serve immediately.

**Per Serving (1½ cups)**

| | |
|---|---|
| Calories: 191 | Fiber: 1 gram |
| Fat: 5 grams | Carbohydrates: 8 grams |
| Protein: 27 grams | Sugar: 4 grams |
| Sodium: 80 milligrams | |

# Spicy, Sweet, and Tangy Barbecue Sauce

**Prep Time:** 5 minutes
**Cook Time:** 10 minutes
**Total Time:** 15 minutes
**Yields 2 cups**

## INGREDIENTS

2 (8-ounce) cans no-salt-added tomato sauce

3 tablespoons apple cider vinegar

2 tablespoons molasses

1 tablespoon honey

1 teaspoon liquid smoke

2 teaspoons onion powder

1½ teaspoons ground cumin

1 teaspoon ground sweet paprika

½ teaspoon garlic powder

½ teaspoon freshly ground black pepper

⅛ teaspoon ground cayenne pepper

Salt-free, fat-free, and absolutely amazing! An authentic-tasting barbecue sauce for all of your grilling, basting, and dipping needs. This is a great recipe to make on a weekend. If stored in an airtight container in the refrigerator, this recipe will keep well for a week. For longer-term storage, seal in a freezer-safe container and thaw before use.

1. Combine ingredients in a saucepan and simmer over medium-low heat for 10 minutes.

2. Remove from heat and pour into a clean lidded jar. Refrigerate until ready to use.

**Per Serving (2 tablespoons)**

Calories: 24
Fat: 0 grams
Protein: 0 grams
Sodium: 4 milligrams

Fiber: 0 grams
Carbohydrates: 5 grams
Sugar: 4 grams

# Chicken Curry with Creamy Tomato Sauce

**Prep Time:** 5 minutes
**Cook Time:** 25 minutes
**Total Time:** 30 minutes
**Serves 4**

## INGREDIENTS

1 pound boneless, skinless chicken breasts

1 teaspoon canola oil

1 large onion, diced

3 cloves garlic, minced

1 tablespoon minced fresh ginger

1 jalapeño pepper, minced

1 (15-ounce) can no-salt-added diced tomatoes

2 tablespoons tomato paste

¾ cup low-sodium chicken or vegetable broth

½ cup nonfat plain yogurt

2 teaspoons salt-free garam masala or curry powder

½ teaspoon ground sweet paprika

¼ teaspoon freshly ground black pepper

¼ cup chopped fresh cilantro

This quick and easy chicken curry tastes terrific and will leave your house smelling glorious. For a less spicy version, simply omit the jalapeño pepper or remove seeds before mincing. Or for added fire, add a second hot pepper and/or increase the curry powder to one tablespoon. Serve over cooked basmati rice for an authentic Indian meal.

1. Wash chicken breasts and pat dry. Cut into bite-sized chunks and set aside.

2. Heat oil in a large sauté pan over medium heat. Add chicken, onion, garlic, and ginger and cook, stirring, for 5 minutes.

3. Add the jalapeño, tomatoes (including juice), tomato paste, broth, yogurt, garam masala, paprika, and black pepper and stir to combine. Bring to a boil.

4. Once boiling, reduce heat to medium-low, cover and simmer, stirring frequently, until chicken is fully cooked, about 20 minutes.

5. Remove from heat. Stir in the cilantro and serve immediately.

**Per Serving (1⅔ cups)**

| | |
|---|---|
| Calories: 189 | Fiber: 1 gram |
| Fat: 3 grams | Carbohydrates: 10 grams |
| Protein: 29 grams | Sugar: 6 grams |
| Sodium: 130 milligrams | |

# Easy Spaghetti and Meatballs

**Prep Time:** 5 minutes
**Cook Time:** 25 minutes
**Total Time:** 30 minutes
**Serves 8**

## INGREDIENTS

1 pound extra-lean ground beef

1 medium onion, grated

2 cloves garlic, grated

1 egg white, beaten

½ cup salt-free bread crumbs

1 tablespoon grated Parmesan cheese

1 teaspoon dried basil

½ teaspoon dried oregano

½ teaspoon dried thyme

Freshly ground black pepper, to taste

2 tablespoons olive oil

2 cups no-salt-added pasta sauce

1 pound dry whole-grain spaghetti

### Love Spaghetti? Try Spaghetti Squash!

Spaghetti squash is a type of winter squash with a firm yellow shell and an inner flesh that shreds into pasta-like strands. To cook spaghetti squash, first slice in half lengthwise and remove the seeds. Place the halves into a microwave-safe bowl. Add ½ cup water, cover, and microwave on high 10–20 minutes, depending upon size. When tender, remove from microwave and shred into strands using a fork.

Who doesn't like spaghetti and meatballs? Here's a simple, delicious, and inexpensive recipe everyone can agree on. As long as you have the ingredients on hand, it's a meal you can whip up anytime. The meatballs also freeze beautifully, so double or triple the recipe, seal leftovers in an airtight container, and keep for a quick meal that's ready when you are.

1. Place ground beef in a mixing bowl and add the grated onion and garlic. Mix together using your hands.

2. Add the egg white, bread crumbs, cheese, and seasonings, and mix thoroughly.

3. To make the meatballs, pinch off 1–2 tablespoons of the meat mixture and roll between your palms to achieve a nice globe. Set the meatball aside and repeat with remaining meat mixture, until you have roughly 24 (2-inch) meatballs.

4. Heat the olive oil in a large sauté pan over medium heat. Add the meatballs and brown on all sides, roughly 3–5 minutes.

5. Once the meatballs have browned, add the pasta sauce, reduce heat to low, cover, and simmer for 20 minutes, stirring or shaking the pan every so often.

6. Bring a stockpot of water to boil over high heat. Once boiling, add the spaghetti and cook according to directions on the package, omitting salt.

7. Drain, then pour the sauce and meatballs over top. Serve immediately.

**Per Serving (1 cup pasta, ¼ cup sauce, and 4 meatballs)**
Calories: 387
Fat: 8 grams
Protein: 23 grams
Sodium: 63 milligrams
Fiber: 4 grams
Carbohydrates: 54 grams
Sugar: 4 grams

# 30-Minute Ground Beef Pizza

Prep Time: 5 minutes
Cook Time: 25 minutes
Total Time: 30 minutes
Serves 4

## INGREDIENTS

1 cup white whole-wheat flour

1 teaspoon all-purpose salt-free seasoning

1 teaspoon salt-free Italian seasoning

½ teaspoon garlic powder

2 egg whites

⅔ cup low-fat milk

½ pound lean ground beef

1 medium onion, chopped

½ cup no-salt-added pasta sauce

2 plum tomatoes, sliced

1 cup sliced mushrooms

1 small bell pepper, diced

3 cloves garlic, minced

¼ cup chopped fresh basil

¼ cup shredded Swiss cheese

¼ cup nonfat ricotta cheese

If you thought "real" pizza was gone from your life, think again! This supremely delicious pizza is flavored with lean ground beef and fresh veggies. Vary toppings according to taste, or add sliced low-sodium olives for a special treat. For those with gluten sensitivities, substitute a wheat-free flour blend. Just be sure to grease the pan extremely well, as gluten-free flours have a tendency to stick.

1. Preheat oven to 450°F. Grease and flour a 12-inch nonstick pizza pan and set aside.

2. Mix the flour, seasonings, and garlic powder in a bowl. Add the egg whites and milk and stir well. Pour batter into the prepared pizza pan, spread to edges, and set aside.

3. Place a large skillet over medium heat. Add the ground beef and onion and cook, stirring, for 5 minutes. Remove from heat and carefully drain any excess fat.

4. Spoon mixture evenly over the batter in the pan. Place pan on middle rack in oven and bake for 15 minutes.

5. Remove pan from oven and spread pasta sauce evenly over pizza. Top with tomatoes, mushrooms, bell pepper, garlic, and chopped basil. Sprinkle the Swiss cheese over the pizza, then dollop evenly with ricotta.

6. Return pan to oven and bake for 5 minutes, until cheese has melted.

7. Remove pizza from oven. Gently remove from pan and cut into 8 slices. Serve immediately.

**Per Serving (2 slices)**
Calories: 302
Fat: 8 grams
Protein: 23 grams
Sodium: 121 milligrams

Fiber: 5 grams
Carbohydrates: 33 grams
Sugar: 6 grams

# Beef Tacos

**Prep Time:** 5 minutes
**Cook Time:** 15 minutes
**Total Time:** 20 minutes
**Serves 6**

## INGREDIENTS

1 pound extra-lean ground beef

1 large onion, chopped

2 cloves garlic, minced

1 (8-ounce) can no-salt-added tomato sauce

2 teaspoons low-sodium Worcestershire sauce

1 tablespoon molasses

1 tablespoon apple cider vinegar

1 tablespoon ground cumin

1 tablespoon ground sweet paprika

½ teaspoon dried red pepper flakes

Freshly ground black pepper, to taste

1 package low-sodium taco shells

¼ cup chopped fresh cilantro

**Low-Sodium Worcestershire Sauce**
Traditional Worcestershire sauce derives its unique taste from salted fermented anchovies, and often contains as much as 65 milligrams of sodium per teaspoon. Fortunately, you can find low-sodium versions both in stores and online. Look for either Lea & Perrins or French's Reduced Sodium Worcestershire Sauce.

This mini fiesta will feed 6 people and makes a great excuse to invite friends over for margaritas—unsalted, of course! Double or triple the filling and freeze for quick meals later in the week or month. Serve the tacos with chopped ripe tomato, lettuce, shredded low-fat, low-sodium cheese, nonfat sour cream, and Holy Guacamole (see recipe in Chapter 5: Snacks and Drinks). Olé!

1. Place the ground beef, onion, and garlic into a sauté pan over medium heat and cook, stirring, until the beef is browned, roughly 3–5 minutes.

2. Once beef is cooked, reduce heat to medium-low and add the tomato sauce, Worcestershire sauce, molasses, vinegar, cumin, paprika, red pepper flakes, and black pepper. Simmer, stirring frequently, about 10 minutes.

3. Heat taco shells according to package directions. Remove from oven and set aside.

4. Remove sauté pan from heat. Stir in cilantro, then divide evenly between the taco shells.

5. If desired, garnish with tomato, lettuce, nonfat sour cream, low-sodium salsa, and guacamole. Serve immediately.

**Per Serving (2 tacos)**

| | |
|---|---|
| Calories: 255 | Fiber: 2 grams |
| Fat: 9 grams | Carbohydrates: 23 grams |
| Protein: 18 grams | Sugar: 4 grams |
| Sodium: 79 milligrams | |

# Cajun-Style Dirty Rice

Prep Time: 5 minutes
Cook Time: 25 minutes
Total Time: 30 minutes
Serves 4

## INGREDIENTS

½ pound extra-lean ground beef

1 large onion, diced

2 medium stalks celery, diced

2 cloves garlic, minced

1 medium bell pepper, diced

1 teaspoon sodium-free beef bouillon granules

1 cup water

2 teaspoons low-sodium Worcestershire sauce

1½ teaspoons dried thyme

1 teaspoon dried basil

½ teaspoon dried marjoram

¼ teaspoon freshly ground black pepper

Pinch ground cayenne pepper

2 scallions, sliced

3 cups cooked long-grain brown rice

This classic Cajun dish has been reworked to be much lower in fat and sodium, but with all the flavor of the original. It makes a wonderful one-skillet supper or side dish. Serve with mixed sautéed veggies and Sweet Corn Muffins (see recipe in Chapter 2: Breakfasts) for a complete and satisfying meal. Adapted from *Prevention's The Healthy Cook*.

1. Place the ground beef, onion, celery, and garlic into a sauté pan over medium heat. Cook until the beef is browned, roughly 5 minutes.

2. Add bell pepper, beef bouillon, water, Worcestershire sauce, herbs, and pepper and stir to combine.

3. Bring to a boil, then reduce heat to low, cover, and simmer for 20 minutes.

4. Remove from heat and stir in the scallions. Add the cooked rice and stir well to combine. Serve immediately.

**Per Serving (1¾ cups)**
Calories: 272
Fat: 4 grams
Protein: 16 grams
Sodium: 92 milligrams

Fiber: 4 grams
Carbohydrates: 41 grams
Sugar: 4 grams

# Quick and Easy Shepherd's Pie

Prep Time: 5 minutes
Cook Time: 25 minutes
Total Time: 30 minutes
Serves 6

## INGREDIENTS

3 cups diced potato

1 pound lean ground beef

1 small onion, diced

3 cloves garlic, minced

1 medium carrot, diced

1 medium stalk celery, diced

1 cup frozen peas

2 tablespoons no-salt-added tomato paste

1 teaspoon dried oregano

½ teaspoon dried basil

½ teaspoon dried thyme

¼ teaspoon freshly ground black pepper

5 tablespoons low-fat milk

2 tablespoons nonfat sour cream

1 tablespoon unsalted butter

1 teaspoon all-purpose salt-free seasoning

1 teaspoon onion powder

½ teaspoon garlic powder

Freshly ground black pepper, to taste

A delicious comfort food at its low-sodium finest, this recipe features flavorful layers of lean ground beef and veggies tucked underneath a crisp blanket of mashed potatoes. Double the recipe when you have extra time and freeze the second pie for a quick meal. Steps like this make healthy living easy and pleasurable, since all you have to do to dig into a delicious, homemade meal is thaw and reheat it!

1. Preheat oven to 450°F. Take out an 8-inch baking dish and set aside.

2. Place diced potato in a saucepan and add enough water to cover by 1 inch. Bring to a boil over high heat, then reduce heat slightly, and continue boiling for 10 minutes.

3. While the potatoes are boiling, heat a large skillet over medium-high heat. Add ground beef, onion, garlic, carrot, and celery, and cook, stirring, for 5 minutes.

4. In the last minute of cooking, stir in the peas, tomato paste, oregano, basil, thyme, and black pepper. Spoon contents into baking dish.

5. Once the potatoes are tender, drain, then mash. Add the remaining ingredients to the mashed potatoes and stir well to combine.

6. Spoon the mashed potatoes over the mixture in the baking dish, then smooth, making sure edges are sealed. Place baking dish on top rack in oven and bake for 10 minutes.

7. Remove from oven and serve immediately.

**Per Serving (1⅔ cups)**
Calories: 280
Fat: 10 grams
Protein: 19 grams
Sodium: 111 milligrams

Fiber: 3 grams
Carbohydrates: 28 grams
Sugar: 11 grams

# Lamb Chops with Rosemary

**Prep Time:** 5 minutes
**Cook Time:** 8 minutes
**Total Time:** 13 minutes
**Serves 4**

## INGREDIENTS

5 cloves garlic, minced
1 tablespoon chopped fresh rosemary
½ teaspoon freshly ground black pepper
1 tablespoon olive oil
1 pound lamb chops

These simple broiled chops make a deliciously elegant dinner any night of the week. To release as much of the essential oil, flavor, and scent as possible, crush and crumble the rosemary leaves between your fingers before adding them. If you don't have fresh rosemary, substitute a teaspoon or two of the dried herb.

1. Adjust oven rack to the top third of the oven. Preheat broiler. Line a baking sheet with foil.

2. Place the garlic, rosemary, pepper, and olive oil into a small bowl and stir well to combine.

3. Place the lamb chops on a baking sheet and brush half of the garlic-rosemary mixture equally between the chops, coating well. Place the sheet beneath broiler and broil 4–5 minutes.

4. Remove from oven and carefully flip over the chops. Divide the remaining garlic-rosemary mixture evenly between the chops and spread to coat. Return pan to oven and broil for another 3 minutes.

5. Remove from oven and serve immediately.

**Per Serving (¼ of the chops)**

| | |
|---|---|
| Calories: 185 | Fiber: 0 grams |
| Fat: 9 grams | Carbohydrates: 1 gram |
| Protein: 23 grams | Sugar: 0 grams |
| Sodium: 73 milligrams | |

# Ginger and Garlic Pork Stir-Fry

**Prep Time:** 5 minutes
**Cook Time:** 10 minutes
**Total Time:** 15 minutes
**Serves 4**

## INGREDIENTS

8 ounces pork tenderloin, sliced thinly

1½ tablespoons minced fresh ginger

3 cloves garlic, minced

2 tablespoons Faux Soy Sauce (see recipe in this chapter)

¾ cup low-sodium vegetable broth

2 teaspoons cornstarch

2 teaspoons sesame oil

1 head bok choy, sliced

½ pound pea pods or sugar snap peas

2 medium carrots, sliced

1 medium red bell pepper, diced

1 small red onion, diced

4 scallions, sliced

Freshly ground black pepper, to taste

Intensely flavorful and speedy to prepare, this low-sodium stir-fry features tender pork loin and crisp veggies in a delectable sauce. If you're unfamiliar with bok choy, it's a type of small cabbage often used in Asian cuisine. The stalks can be sliced much like celery. If you can't find it locally, feel free to use another vegetable such as broccoli.

1. Place pork into a mixing bowl, add the minced ginger, garlic, and faux soy sauce and stir well to coat. Set aside.

2. Measure the broth and cornstarch into a second bowl and whisk well to combine. Set aside.

3. Heat the oil in a wok over medium heat. Add the bok choy, pea pods, carrots, bell pepper, and onion and cook, stirring, for 5 minutes.

4. Add the pork mixture and cook, stirring, for 3 minutes.

5. Add the broth mixture and cook, stirring, until sauce thickens, roughly 30 seconds to 1 minute.

6. Remove from heat. Stir in the sliced scallions and season to taste with freshly ground black pepper. Serve immediately.

**Per Serving (1½ cups)**

| | |
|---|---|
| Calories: 180 | Fiber: 5 grams |
| Fat: 4 grams | Carbohydrates: 20 grams |
| Protein: 17 grams | Sugar: 10 grams |
| Sodium: 323 grams | |

# Asian-Inspired Mini Meatloaves with Salt-Free Hoisin Glaze

**Prep Time:** 5 minutes
**Cook Time:** 25 minutes
**Total Time:** 30 minutes
**Serves 4**

## INGREDIENTS

½ pound lean ground pork

1 medium red bell pepper, diced

¾ cup shelled edamame

3 scallions, sliced

3 cloves garlic, minced

1 tablespoon minced fresh ginger

1 egg white

⅓ cup salt-free bread crumbs

½ teaspoon ground 5-spice powder

¼ teaspoon ground white pepper

3 tablespoons Faux Soy Sauce, divided (see recipe in this chapter)

1 tablespoon salt-free tomato paste

These tasty little loaves are loaded with veggies and the tantalizing flavors of ginger, garlic, and 5-spice powder. After baking, the loaves positively glisten with caramelized flavor! An easy and authentic-tasting salt-free hoisin glaze is prepared from Faux Soy Sauce and tomato paste. The 5-spice powder is a special Asian blend available at many supermarkets. If you can't find it, use ½ teaspoon ground cinnamon and a dash of ground cloves instead.

1. Preheat oven to 400°F. Spray 4 cups of a jumbo muffin tin lightly with oil and set aside.

2. Place the pork, bell pepper, edamame, scallions, garlic, ginger, egg white, bread crumbs, 5-spice powder, and pepper into a bowl. Add 1 tablespoon faux soy sauce and mix together using your hands.

3. Divide mixture into 4 equal portions and press into the prepared muffin tin cups.

4. Measure the remaining 2 tablespoons faux soy sauce and the tomato paste into a small bowl and stir until smooth. Brush onto the tops of the meatloaves, dividing evenly.

5. Place muffin tin on middle rack in oven and bake for 25 minutes.

6. Remove from oven, gently run a knife around the sides of each loaf, and remove from tin. Serve immediately.

**Per Serving (1 mini meatloaf)**
Calories: 205
Fat: 6 grams
Protein: 17 grams
Sodium: 56 milligrams

Fiber: 3 grams
Carbohydrates: 20 grams
Sugar: 7 grams

# Barbecue Pizza with Ground Pork, Peppers, and Pineapple

**Prep Time:** 5 minutes
**Cook Time:** 25 minutes
**Total Time:** 30 minutes
**Serves 4**

## INGREDIENTS

1 cup white whole-wheat flour

1 teaspoon all-purpose salt-free seasoning

1 teaspoon salt-free Italian seasoning

½ teaspoon garlic powder

2 egg whites

⅔ cup low-fat milk

½ pound lean ground pork

2 teaspoons salt-free chili seasoning

1 medium red onion, chopped

½ cup Spicy, Sweet, and Tangy Barbecue Sauce (see recipe in this chapter)

1 cup diced fresh pineapple

1 small red bell pepper, diced

1 jalapeño pepper, minced

3 cloves garlic, minced

2 tablespoons chopped fresh cilantro

¼ cup shredded Swiss cheese

This healthy take on Hawaiian pizza has so much flavor, you won't believe it's salt-free! The tangy home-made barbecue sauce comes together in just 10 minutes. For ease, you may want to make the sauce ahead of time and refrigerate until ready to cook. If you don't care for spice, omit the jalapeño or seed the pepper before mincing to reduce its kick.

1. Preheat oven to 450°F. Grease and flour a 12-inch nonstick pizza pan and set aside.

2. Place the flour, seasonings, and garlic powder into a mixing bowl and whisk well to combine.

3. Add the egg whites and milk and stir well. Pour batter into the prepared pizza pan, spread to edges, and set aside.

4. Place a large skillet over medium heat. Add the ground pork, salt-free chili seasoning, and onion and cook, stirring, for 5 minutes. Remove from heat and carefully drain any excess fat.

5. Spoon mixture evenly over the batter in the pan. Place pan on middle rack in oven and bake for 15 minutes.

6. Remove pan from oven, spread the barbecue sauce evenly over pizza, then top with pineapple, peppers, garlic, and chopped cilantro. Sprinkle the Swiss cheese over the pizza.

continued on next page

7. Return pan to oven and bake for 5 minutes, until cheese has melted.

8. Remove pizza from oven. Gently remove from pan and cut into 8 slices. Serve immediately.

**Per Serving (2 slices)**
Calories: 306
Fat: 7 grams
Protein: 21 grams
Sodium: 98 milligrams

Fiber: 5 grams
Carbohydrates: 39 grams
Sugar: 12 grams

# Southwestern Salmon

**Prep Time:** 5 minutes
**Cook Time:** 7 minutes
**Total Time:** 12 minutes
**Serves 4**

## INGREDIENTS

1 teaspoon dried cilantro

1 teaspoon ground cumin

1 teaspoon ground paprika

½ teaspoon freshly ground black pepper

½ teaspoon ground coriander

⅛ teaspoon ground cayenne pepper

1 pound boneless salmon fillet

### Savory Broiled Salmon

In a small bowl, combine 1 teaspoon dried marjoram, ½ teaspoon each dried savory and ground white pepper, and ¼ teaspoon each dried thyme, ground rosemary, and garlic powder. Gently rub the mixture into a 1-pound boneless salmon fillet, then broil 7–8 minutes. The rub adds an extra jolt of flavor to an already tasty fish, and the broiling process renders the flesh crisp outside and juicy within.

The colorful seasoning mix in this recipe is as pretty as it is flavorful, and the resulting fish is crisp, juicy, and delicious. Pair the salmon with Southwestern Rice Pilaf (see recipe in Chapter 6: Appetizers and Side Dishes) for a spectacular salt-free meal. Another version of this recipe—with savory herbs instead of spice—is shown in the sidebar.

1. Move a rack to the top of the oven and preheat broiler. Spray a baking sheet lightly with oil and set aside.

2. Place the seasonings into a small bowl and mix well to combine.

3. Sprinkle the spice mixture over the salmon fillet and gently rub the mixture into the fish. Place the fillet on the prepared baking sheet.

4. Place the sheet on the top rack in the oven and broil for about 7 minutes; 1–2 minutes less for thin fillets, a little longer for thicker fillets. When cooked fully, salmon will be opaque and flake easily.

5. Remove sheet from oven, slice salmon into 4 portions, and serve immediately.

**Per Serving (¼ of the fillet)**

| | |
|---|---|
| Calories: 171 | Fiber: 0 grams |
| Fat: 8 grams | Carbohydrates: 0 grams |
| Protein: 22 grams | Sugar: 0 grams |
| Sodium: 50 milligrams | |

# Baked Tuna Cakes

**Prep Time:** 10 minutes
**Cook Time:** 15 minutes
**Total Time:** 25 minutes
**Serves 4**

## INGREDIENTS

2 (5-ounce) cans no-salt-added tuna, in water

1 small carrot, shredded

1 small stalk celery, finely diced

1 shallot, minced

2 cloves garlic, minced

1 egg white

¼ cup salt-free bread crumbs

2 tablespoons Salt-Free Mayonnaise (see Chapter 3: Salads and Dressings)

½ teaspoon dried dill

½ teaspoon dried thyme

¼ teaspoon ground rosemary

Freshly ground black pepper, to taste

This moist and healthy twist on crab cakes is accented with veggies and a crisp oven-fried crust. Salt-free tuna is readily available at most supermarkets. If you can't find it, you can substitute regular canned tuna, but rinse well in a fine mesh sieve to remove as much sodium as possible. Use salt-free canned salmon for another take on this recipe.

1. Preheat oven to 400°F. Spray a baking sheet lightly with oil and set aside.

2. Drain the tuna and place in a mixing bowl. Add remaining ingredients and stir well to combine.

3. Shape mixture into 4 equal patties and place on the prepared baking sheet.

4. Place baking sheet on middle rack in oven and bake 10 minutes. Remove from oven, gently flip, and bake 5 minutes more. Remove from oven and serve immediately.

**Per Serving (1 cake)**
Calories: 163
Fat: 5 grams
Protein: 20 grams
Sodium: 66 milligrams
Fiber: 1 gram
Carbohydrates: 8 grams
Sugar: 1 gram

# Pasta with Cherry Tomatoes, Tuna, and Lemon

**Prep Time:** 10 minutes
**Cook Time:** 15 minutes
**Total Time:** 25 minutes
**Serves 8**

## INGREDIENTS

1 pound dry pasta (your choice)

3 tablespoons unsalted butter

4 cups ripe cherry tomatoes, halved

2 cloves garlic, minced

1 (5-ounce) can no-salt-added tuna, in water

Juice and grated zest of 1 fresh lemon

3 tablespoons grated Parmesan cheese

1 tablespoon chopped fresh parsley

Freshly ground black pepper, to taste

A hearty dish that's also light, sunny, and refreshing, this pasta recipe is ready in just 25 minutes! It tastes great the first day, but even better the next, so feel free to double the recipe for a fabulous leftover meal. For an even more wholesome meal, pair the pasta with steamed asparagus or fresh green beans sautéed with garlic and slivered almonds.

1. Cook pasta according to package directions, omitting salt. Drain, leaving a tiny bit of water in the bottom of the pot.

2. Melt the butter in a sauté pan over medium heat. Add the tomatoes and garlic and cook, stirring, for 3 minutes.

3. Add the tuna and lemon juice and cook, stirring, for 2 minutes.

4. Remove pan from heat and add contents to the pot of pasta, along with the lemon zest and Parmesan. Sprinkle with the chopped parsley and season to taste with freshly ground black pepper.

5. Serve immediately.

**Per Serving (1⅔ cups)**

| | |
|---|---|
| Calories: 308 | Fiber: 3 grams |
| Fat: 6 grams | Carbohydrates: 47 grams |
| Protein: 13 grams | Sugar: 3 grams |
| Sodium: 44 milligrams | |

# Tuna Noodle Casserole

**Prep Time:** 5 minutes
**Cook Time:** 25 minutes
**Total Time:** 30 minutes
**Serves 6**

## INGREDIENTS

2 teaspoons canola oil

10 ounces fresh mushrooms, sliced

2 medium carrots, diced

2 medium stalks celery, diced

1 medium bell pepper, diced

1 medium onion, diced

4 cloves garlic, minced

1 pound whole-grain yolkless egg noodles, cooked

2 (6-ounce) cans no-salt-added tuna in water, drained

1 cup nonfat sour cream

½ cup shredded Swiss cheese

2 teaspoons all-purpose salt-free seasoning

½ teaspoon dried herbes de Provence

Freshly ground black pepper, to taste

Classic American comfort food at its best! This is a great make-ahead meal: assemble in the morning or the night before, cover, refrigerate, then pop into the oven when you're ready to eat. Nonfat plain yogurt may be used instead of sour cream. If you don't have herbes de Provence, substitute a ½ teaspoon of dried dill or thyme instead.

1. Preheat oven to 375°F. Take out a 3-quart baking dish, spray lightly with oil, and set aside.

2. Heat oil in a large sauté pan over medium heat. Add mushrooms, carrots, celery, bell pepper, onion, and garlic and cook, stirring, for 5 minutes. Remove from heat.

3. Add the cooked noodles, along with the remaining ingredients, and stir well to combine.

4. Pour mixture into the prepared baking dish and cover with lid or aluminum foil. Place on middle rack in oven and bake for 20 minutes.

5. Remove from oven and serve immediately.

**Per Serving (2 cups)**
Calories: 434
Fat: 9 grams
Protein: 29 grams
Sodium: 137 milligrams

Fiber: 4 grams
Carbohydrates: 55 grams
Sugar: 4 grams

# Healthy Fish and Chips

## INGREDIENTS

2 tablespoons unbleached all-purpose flour

2 tablespoons white whole-wheat flour

Freshly ground black pepper, to taste

2 egg whites

2 cups salt-free bread crumbs or panko

1 tablespoon dried herbs (a single herb or mix of favorites, such as parsley, dill, thyme, etc.)

1 pound white-fleshed fish (4 fillets)

4 large potatoes, scrubbed

3 tablespoons olive oil

Freshly ground black pepper, to taste

### Low-Sodium Tartar Sauce

Whip up a batch of low-sodium tartar sauce in minutes by combining ¼ cup Salt-Free Mayonnaise (see Chapter 3: Salads and Dressings) with a tablespoon of salt-free pickle relish. Use immediately or cover and refrigerate until serving. Salt-free pickle relish is sold at select stores and online at http://healthyheartmarket.com.

This healthy, salt-free version of the beloved coastal dinner is baked rather than fried. Choose your favorite white-fleshed fish, such as haddock, pollock, or cod. Serve with lemon wedges, malt vinegar, and salt-free ketchup. For a different variation, substitute sweet potatoes for all or half of the regular potatoes. Adapted from *I'm Hungry, Let's Cook*.

1. Preheat oven to 425°F. Take out a large baking sheet, cover with aluminum foil, and set aside.

2. Measure the flours into a wide shallow bowl, add freshly ground black pepper to taste, and whisk to combine.

3. Place the egg whites into a second shallow bowl.

4. Measure the bread crumbs into a large plastic bag. Add dried herbs, seal bag, and shake well to combine.

5. Cut the fish fillets in half, yielding 8 pieces total. Dredge each fillet completely in the seasoned flour, then dip in egg whites, coating completely.

6. Place a moistened fillet into the plastic bag, seal, and shake gently to coat. Once the fillet is entirely coated in bread crumbs, carefully remove from bag and place on the prepared baking sheet. Repeat process with the remaining fillets until all pieces are battered. Place the tray of fish in the refrigerator.

7. Place a piece of parchment paper on a baking sheet. Cut each potato into 8 equal wedges. Arrange the wedges on the baking sheet and brush both sides lightly with olive oil. Season to taste with freshly ground black pepper.

continued on next page

8. Place baking sheet on middle rack in oven and bake for 15 minutes. Remove from oven and flip potatoes over. Return to oven.

9. Remove the fish from the refrigerator and place on the top rack in oven. Bake potatoes and fish for 10 minutes, until both are crispy and brown.

10. Remove from oven and serve immediately.

**Per Serving (2 pieces fish and 8 potato wedges)**

| | |
|---|---|
| Calories: 534 | Fiber: 5 grams |
| Fat: 13 grams | Carbohydrates: 65 grams |
| Protein: 38 grams | Sugar: 5 grams |
| Sodium: 142 milligrams | |

# Shrimp Creole

**Prep Time:** 10 minutes
**Cook Time:** 20 minutes
**Total Time:** 30 minutes
**Serves 6**

## INGREDIENTS

2 teaspoons canola oil

1 medium onion, thinly sliced

1 medium bell pepper, thinly sliced

2 medium stalks celery, thinly sliced

3 cloves garlic, minced

2 (15-ounce) cans no-salt-added diced tomatoes

1 (8-ounce) can no-salt-added tomato sauce

⅓ cup white wine

½ teaspoon apple cider vinegar

2 bay leaves

2 teaspoons salt-free chili seasoning

1 teaspoon ground sweet paprika

½ teaspoon freshly ground black pepper

⅛ teaspoon ground cayenne pepper

1 pound peeled shrimp, tails removed

### The Skinny on Shrimp

Shrimp are fairly high in sodium naturally, with roughly 160 milligrams per 3-ounce serving, so they should be consumed carefully. Shrimp come in a variety of sizes, from miniscule to extra colossal, and are typically sold by weight and size; for instance, a pound of large shrimp contains roughly 30–35 pieces. Most shrimp consumed in the United States have been processed to some degree and may have added salt. Read package labels carefully and buy fresh, unprocessed shrimp whenever possible.

Amazing flavor with none of the salt! This spicy and beautiful shrimp dish is made for special occasions, but is quick and easy enough to enjoy anytime. Remove as much excess sodium from the shrimp by soaking them in cold water, and rinsing repeatedly. Serve over cooked rice with lemon wedges, and a nice green salad on the side.

1. Heat oil in a large sauté pan over medium heat. Add the onion, bell pepper, celery, and garlic and cook, stirring, for 5 minutes.

2. Add the remaining ingredients except shrimp and stir well to combine. Simmer for 10 minutes, stirring frequently. Cover and reduce heat to medium-low if sauce begins to splatter.

3. Stir in the shrimp and simmer for 5 minutes.

4. Remove from heat and remove bay leaves from pan. Serve immediately.

**Per Serving (1⅔ cups)**
Calories: 152
Fat: 3 grams
Protein: 17 grams
Sodium: 136 milligrams
Fiber: 2 grams
Carbohydrates: 11 grams
Sugar: 6 grams

# CHAPTER 8

# Vegan and Vegetarian Dishes

# 30-Minute Vegetarian Pizza

**Prep Time:** 5 minutes
**Cook Time:** 25 minutes
**Total Time:** 30 minutes
**Serves 4**

## INGREDIENTS

1 cup white whole-wheat flour

1 teaspoon all-purpose salt-free seasoning

1 teaspoon salt-free Italian seasoning

½ teaspoon garlic powder

2 egg whites

⅔ cup low-fat milk

2 teaspoons olive oil

1 small eggplant, peeled and diced

1 medium onion, diced

½ cup no-salt-added pasta sauce

1 small bell pepper, diced

1 small tomato, diced

1 cup sliced mushrooms

½ cup chopped fresh broccoli

2 cloves garlic, minced

2 tablespoons chopped fresh basil

½ cup shredded Swiss cheese

### Easy Greasing

The simplest way to grease and flour a pizza pan is by using an oil cooking spray. Spray pan lightly with oil, add 1–2 tablespoons flour, then tap pan and tilt to disperse the flour. After surface is evenly coated, tip pan over the sink, compost bin, or trashcan and tap lightly to remove excess flour.

In one word: *yum*! Make it vegan by substituting nutritional yeast flakes, egg replacement powder, and nondairy milk for the animal products. An equally good gluten-free version can be made using brown rice flour. However, gluten-free crusts have a tendency to stick, so make sure the pan is really well oiled and floured.

1. Preheat oven to 450°F. Grease and flour a 12-inch nonstick pizza pan and set aside.

2. Place the flour and seasonings, including garlic powder, into a mixing bowl and whisk well to combine. Add the egg whites and milk and stir well. Pour batter into the prepared pizza pan, spread to edges, and set aside.

3. Place a large skillet over medium heat. Add the diced eggplant and onion and cook, stirring, for 5 minutes.

4. Remove from heat and spoon mixture evenly over the batter in the pan. Place pan on middle rack in oven and bake for 15 minutes.

5. Remove pan from oven and spread pasta sauce evenly over crust. Top pizza with bell pepper, tomato, mushrooms, broccoli, garlic, and basil. Sprinkle the Swiss cheese evenly over top.

6. Return pan to oven and bake 5 minutes, until cheese has melted.

7. Remove pan from oven. Gently remove pizza from pan and cut into 8 slices. Serve immediately.

**Per Serving (2 slices)**
Calories: 242
Fat: 7 grams
Protein: 13 grams
Sodium: 82 milligrams

Fiber: 6 grams
Carbohydrates: 34 grams
Sugar: 7 grams

# Vegetable Fried Rice

Prep Time: 10 minutes
Cook Time: 10 minutes
Total Time: 20 minutes
Serves 4

## INGREDIENTS

1 tablespoon sesame oil

1 medium onion, diced

3 medium carrots, sliced

1 bunch fresh broccoli, cut into florets

2 cups sugar snap peas or snow pea pods

3 cloves garlic, minced

1 tablespoon minced fresh ginger

4 cups cooked brown rice

1 tablespoon low-sodium soy sauce

½ teaspoon freshly ground black pepper

Thanks to garlic, ginger, and low-sodium soy sauce, this vegetarian fried rice has authentic taste with very little salt. Add tofu and chopped cashews for added heft and protein. Or for a deliciously sweet variation, swap the broccoli out for 1¼ cups (or a 15-ounce can) of diced pineapple.

1. Heat oil in a wok over medium heat. When oil begins to sizzle, add vegetables, garlic, and ginger and cook, stirring, for 5 minutes.

2. Add rice, soy sauce, and black pepper and cook, stirring, another 5 minutes.

3. Remove from heat and serve immediately.

**Per Serving (2 cups)**

| | |
|---|---|
| Calories: 341 | Fiber: 9 grams |
| Fat: 6 grams | Carbohydrates: 64 grams |
| Protein: 10 grams | Sugar: 8 grams |
| Sodium: 94 milligrams | |

# Coconut Collards with Sweet Potatoes and Black Beans

Prep Time: 7 minutes
Cook Time: 23 minutes
Total Time: 30 minutes
Serves 8

## INGREDIENTS

1 tablespoon olive oil (optional, see note in steps)

1 medium onion, chopped

4 cloves garlic, minced

2 medium carrots, sliced

2 medium stalks celery, sliced

1 medium red bell pepper, diced

2 medium sweet potatoes, peeled and cubed

1 pound collard greens, chopped

1 (15-ounce) can no-salt-added diced tomatoes, with juice

1 (15-ounce) can light coconut milk, shaken well

1 (15-ounce) can no-salt-added black beans, drained and rinsed

4 tablespoons no-salt-added tomato paste

1 tablespoon Thai Red Curry Paste

Juice of 2 fresh limes

1½ teaspoons ground cumin

1½ teaspoons ground sweet paprika

¼ teaspoon ground allspice

Freshly ground black pepper, to taste

### Love Your Body, Love Your Collards!

Not only are collards high in fiber, vitamin A, vitamin C, and calcium, they're also considered to be the very best vegetable for naturally lowering blood pressure, and they also protect against cancer. Bonus? Collards are abundant and inexpensive! So you'll never have to burn a hole through your wallet to put your health first.

Talk about fantastic flavor! The collards are bathed with a subtle sweetness from the light coconut milk, sweet potatoes, carrots, and tomatoes. And a citrus kick from the lime juice and curry paste lends the perfect finish. The combination is so seriously stupendous, you won't believe it's low sodium! A note about Thai Red Curry Paste: Although this product does contain salt, when used sparingly it lends tremendous depth of flavor. Thai Red Curry Paste is sold at Asian groceries and in the "international aisle" of most supermarkets. Buy the lowest-sodium brand you can find.

1. Measure the olive oil into a stockpot, or if you prefer, coat bottom of pan with a thin layer of water. Place pot over medium heat. Add the onion, garlic, carrots, celery, bell pepper, and sweet potatoes and cook, stirring, 3 minutes.

2. Add the remaining ingredients and stir well to combine. Cover and simmer over medium heat, stirring frequently, 10 minutes.

3. Reduce heat to medium-low to low, and continue to simmer, stirring frequently, 5–10 minutes more. Keep checking to make sure the mixture isn't cooking too fast or beginning to stick and burn. Dish is ready when the sweet potatoes are fork tender.

4. Remove from heat and serve immediately over cooked rice, quinoa, or your favorite whole grain.

Per Serving (2 cups)
Calories: 208
Fat: 6 grams
Protein: 8 grams
Sodium: 102 milligrams

Fiber: 9 grams
Carbohydrates: 30 grams
Sugar: 6 grams

# Zucchini Cakes

**Prep Time:** 10 minutes
**Cook Time:** 20 minutes
**Total Time:** 30 minutes
**Serves 4**

## INGREDIENTS

1 medium zucchini, shredded (with skin)

1 small red onion, finely diced

1 egg white

¾ cup salt-free bread crumbs

2 teaspoons salt-free all-purpose seasoning

Freshly ground black pepper, to taste

### Homemade Horseradish Sauce
Combine 2 tablespoons store-bought horseradish with ¼ cup nonfat sour cream. Add 1–2 tablespoons of chopped fresh herbs, such as dill or chives, a minced clove of garlic, and freshly ground black pepper to taste. Use immediately or cover and refrigerate until ready to serve.

Yummy, versatile, and under 20 mg of sodium, zucchini is a great vegetable for those on the DASH diet. But when you're inundated with the stuff, what do you do with it? These scrumptious oven-baked patties are a perfect way to use some of your garden surplus. Garnish with homemade horseradish sauce (see recipe in sidebar) or salt-free ketchup.

1. Preheat oven to 400°F. Spray a baking sheet lightly with oil and set aside.

2. Press shredded zucchini gently between paper towels to remove excess liquid.

3. In a large bowl, combine zucchini, onion, egg white, bread crumbs, seasoning, and black pepper. Mix well.

4. Shape mixture into patties and place on the prepared baking sheet.

5. Place baking sheet on middle rack in oven and bake for 10 minutes. Gently flip patties and return to oven to bake for another 10 minutes.

6. Remove from oven and serve immediately.

**Per Serving (1 cake)**

Calories: 94

Fat: 1 gram

Protein: 4 grams

Sodium: 22 milligrams

Fiber: 2 grams

Carbohydrates: 19 grams

Sugar: 2 grams

# Sesame Tofu with Sautéed Green Beans

**Prep Time:** 5 minutes
**Cook Time:** 25 minutes
**Total Time:** 30 minutes
**Serves 4**

## INGREDIENTS

1 pound extra-firm water-packed tofu

1 tablespoon plus 1 teaspoon sesame oil, divided

2 tablespoons toasted sesame seeds

Freshly ground black pepper, to taste

1 pound fresh green beans

1 medium red onion, diced

3 cloves garlic, minced

1 tablespoon minced fresh ginger

Bursting with flavor, this vegan dish is one you won't want to pass up! Be sure to use extra-firm water-packed tofu—the kind sold in the refrigerator case, *not* the silken shelf-stable variety. The baked tofu is toothsome and dense, and the sautéed green beans have an irresistible crunch. It's a meal you can sink your teeth into, literally!

1. Preheat oven to 450°F. Spray a baking sheet lightly with oil and set aside.

2. Drain the tofu and press gently between paper towels to remove excess water.

3. Cut the tofu crosswise into about 24 equal bite-sized pieces. Place tofu in a bowl, add 1 tablespoon sesame oil and, using your hands, toss gently to coat. Arrange tofu on the prepared baking sheet and sprinkle evenly with sesame seeds and freshly ground pepper, to taste.

4. Place baking sheet on middle rack in oven and bake for 15–20 minutes, until tofu is firm and golden brown. Turn over the tofu once, halfway through cooking time.

5. While tofu is baking, wash and trim beans, then cut into roughly 2-inch pieces.

6. Heat 1 teaspoon of sesame oil in a sauté pan over medium heat. Add the onion, garlic, and ginger and sauté for 2 minutes.

7. Add the beans and sauté for 5–8 minutes, until tender-crisp.

continued on next page

8. When tofu is ready, remove from oven and add to the mixture in sauté pan. Stir to coat, season to taste with freshly ground black pepper, and serve immediately.

**Per Serving (1½ cups)**

Calories: 238

Fat: 12 grams

Protein: 15 grams

Sodium: 20 milligrams

Fiber: 6 grams

Carbohydrates: 19 grams

Sugar: 6 grams

# Mushroom and Eggplant Curry

**Prep Time:** 10 minutes
**Cook Time:** 16 minutes
**Total Time:** 26 minutes
**Serves 4**

## INGREDIENTS

1 medium eggplant

1 teaspoon olive oil

1 medium red onion, diced

1 tablespoon minced fresh ginger

3 cloves garlic, minced

8 ounces white mushrooms, sliced

1 cup low-sodium vegetable broth

1 (15-ounce) can no-salt-added diced tomatoes

2½ teaspoons salt-free curry powder

½ teaspoon freshly ground black pepper

¼ cup chopped fresh cilantro

A salt-free curry that's brimming over with taste. The mushrooms and eggplant in this delicious dish are so wholesome and hearty that they'll keep you feeling full for hours! Serve over cooked rice or quinoa for an even tastier meal. For a spicier version, add a minced hot pepper, dash of chili powder or red pepper flakes, or a little extra curry powder.

1. Peel eggplant and cut into 1-inch cubes. Set aside.

2. Heat olive oil in a large skillet or sauté pan over medium heat. Add the onion, ginger, and garlic and sauté for 2 minutes.

3. Add eggplant and mushrooms and cook, stirring, for 3 minutes.

4. Add broth and cook for 1 minute, stirring and scraping to get all of the brown bits off the bottom of the pan.

5. Add tomatoes (including liquid) and curry powder and stir well to combine. Reduce heat to low, cover, and simmer for 10 minutes, stirring once or twice.

6. Remove from heat. Stir in ground pepper and cilantro. Serve immediately.

**Per Serving (1½ cups)**

Calories: 67
Fat: 2 grams
Protein: 3 grams
Sodium: 50 milligrams

Fiber: 3 grams
Carbohydrates: 12 grams
Sugar: 4 grams

# Amazing Veggie Casserole

**Prep Time:** 5 minutes
**Cook Time:** 25 minutes
**Total Time:** 30 minutes
**Serves 8**

## INGREDIENTS

2 teaspoons olive oil

2 medium onions, sliced thinly

½ medium head green cabbage, sliced

1 pound kale, leaves only, chopped

3 medium carrots, sliced into thin sticks

½ cup low-sodium vegetable broth or water

2 tablespoons low-sodium soy sauce

### TOPPING

1½ cups salt-free bread crumbs

8 ounces extra-firm tofu

¼ cup chopped walnuts

2 garlic cloves

2 tablespoons olive oil

2 teaspoons dried basil

1½ teaspoons dried oregano

1 teaspoon ground sweet paprika

### Walnut Facts

Walnuts have a wonderfully nutty flavor that complements everything from baked goods to salads to entrées. They're rich in monounsaturated fats and omega-3 fatty acids, manganese, and copper, and have been shown to prevent cardiovascular disease, lower cholesterol, and inhibit certain types of cancer.

This recipe makes great use of some of the healthiest and least expensive veggies: carrots, onions, cabbage, and kale. Best of all, they're abundantly available year round. Sandwiched under a crust of crumbled tofu, bread crumbs, and chopped nuts, it's an irresistible casserole with tons of taste and texture, and it's super low in sodium! Adapted from *Gourmet* magazine.

1. Preheat oven to 350°F. Take out a 9" × 13" baking dish and set aside.

2. Heat olive oil in a large sauté pan over medium heat. Add onion, cabbage, kale, carrots, broth, and soy sauce. Cover the pan and cook, stirring occasionally, for 10 minutes. Transfer contents to the baking pan and set aside.

3. To make the topping, measure remaining ingredients into a food processor and pulse to combine. Sprinkle over vegetables in baking dish.

4. Place dish on middle rack in oven and bake, uncovered, until topping is golden brown and vegetables are heated through, about 15 minutes.

5. Remove from oven and serve immediately.

**Per Serving (2 cups)**

| | |
|---|---|
| Calories: 238 | Fiber: 6 grams |
| Fat: 9 grams | Carbohydrates: 33 grams |
| Protein: 10 grams | Sugar: 6 grams |
| Sodium: 69 milligrams | |

# Asparagus, Swiss, and Ricotta Frittata

**Prep Time:** 5 minutes
**Cook Time:** 15 minutes
**Total Time:** 20 minutes
**Serves 4**

## INGREDIENTS

8 stalks fresh asparagus

1 shallot, finely diced

1¼ cups liquid egg replacement (e.g., Egg Beaters)

¼ cup Roasted Red Peppers, sliced (see recipe in Chapter 6: Appetizers and Side Dishes)

¼ cup shredded Swiss cheese

1 tablespoon nonfat ricotta cheese

All-purpose salt-free seasoning, to taste

Freshly ground black pepper, to taste

Frittatas are impressive, yet ridiculously easy to make. Liquid egg replacement is used instead of whole eggs because it's so much lower in cholesterol and fat. Liquid egg replacement products, such as Egg Beaters, are stocked alongside the eggs in most supermarkets. If you don't have time to roast the red peppers, simply slice and sauté them for 5 minutes, or until tender.

1. Position rack at top of oven and preheat to 450°F.

2. Trim the asparagus and cut into thirds. Place into the steamer basket of a pot or appliance and steam over high heat for 5 minutes.

3. Spray an ovenproof skillet with cooking oil. Place over medium heat, add shallot, and sauté for 2 minutes.

4. Add liquid egg replacement to skillet and remove from heat.

5. Top with the steamed asparagus, red peppers, and Swiss cheese. Dollop ricotta over top and season with salt-free seasoning and freshly ground black pepper, to taste.

6. Place skillet on top rack in oven and bake for 10 minutes.

7. Remove from oven. Slide a heatproof spatula around and under frittata to loosen. Remove and cut into wedges. Serve immediately.

**Per Serving (¼ of the frittata)**

| | |
|---|---|
| Calories: 112 | Fiber: 1 gram |
| Fat: 4 grams | Carbohydrates: 4 grams |
| Protein: 13 grams | Sugar: 2 grams |
| Sodium: 161 milligrams | |

# Tofu Stroganoff

**Prep Time:** 12 minutes
**Cook Time:** 18 minutes
**Total Time:** 30 minutes
**Serves 6**

## INGREDIENTS

1 pound wide yolkless egg noodles

1 pound extra-firm tofu

4 teaspoons olive oil, divided

1 large onion, diced

4 cloves garlic, minced

3 cups sliced baby bella mushrooms

¼ cup sliced fresh chives

½ teaspoon freshly ground black pepper

¾ cup nonfat sour cream

3 tablespoons low-sodium soy sauce

If you like the combination of creamy sauce, mushrooms, and noodles found in classic Beef Stroganoff, you'll love this updated salt-free version made with tofu. A yummy vegan version can be made by substituting homemade "vegan sour cream" for the nonfat sour cream: Purée a package of silken tofu along with a tablespoon of olive oil, 1½ tablespoons lemon juice, ½ tablespoon apple cider vinegar, 1 teaspoon agave nectar, and 2 teaspoons all-purpose salt-free seasoning. Store leftover "sour cream" in a clean lidded jar in the refrigerator; use within 1 week. Adapted from *Vegetarian Times* magazine.

1. Cook noodles according to package directions, omitting salt. Drain and set aside.

2. Drain tofu and gently press between paper towels to remove as much liquid as possible.

3. Slice tofu into long strips, about 3" long × ¾" wide × ½" in height. Set aside.

4. Heat 2 teaspoons of the olive oil in a sauté pan over medium heat. Add onion, garlic, and mushrooms and cook, stirring, for 8 minutes.

5. Add chives and pepper and stir. Remove mixture from pan and set aside.

6. Return pan to medium heat and add remaining 2 teaspoons of olive oil. Add tofu and cook until golden brown, about 8 minutes.

7. Return the mushroom mixture to the pan, add sour cream and soy sauce, and stir gently. Cook 2 minutes.

continued on next page

8. Remove from heat and spoon over egg noodles (or eggless noodles, if vegan). Serve immediately.

**Per Serving (2 cups)**
Calories: 432
Fat: 12 grams
Protein: 20 grams
Sodium: 62 milligrams

Fiber: 5 grams
Carbohydrates: 59 grams
Sugar: 4 grams

# Spicy Red Lentil Dal with Vegetables

**Prep Time:** 5 minutes
**Cook Time:** 25 minutes
**Total Time:** 30 minutes
**Serves 6**

## INGREDIENTS

1 medium onion, diced

4 cloves garlic, minced

2 tablespoons minced fresh ginger

1 hot pepper, your choice

2 teaspoons canola oil

1½ teaspoons mustard seeds

1 tablespoon salt-free garam masala or curry powder

1½ cups red lentils, rinsed well

½ head cauliflower, broken into florets

4 medium carrots, cut into 1-inch pieces

2 large potatoes, cut into 1-inch chunks

1 teaspoon ground turmeric

6 cups water

¾ cup chopped fresh cilantro

Freshly ground black pepper, to taste

This filling vegan main course is a snap to prepare and sings with the mingling flavors of ginger, garlic, and cilantro. If you dislike cilantro, try substituting another leafy green or herb, like chopped baby spinach, kale, or parsley. If you prefer less heat, simply omit the chili pepper. Adapted from *Fine Cooking*.

1. Place the onion, garlic, ginger, and hot pepper into a food processor and pulse briefly to chop. Set aside.

2. Heat the oil in a stockpot over medium heat. When hot, add the mustard seeds. When the seeds begin to pop, stir in the garam masala or curry powder, along with the onion mixture, lentils, cauliflower, carrots, potatoes, turmeric, and water.

3. Raise heat slightly and bring to a boil. Once boiling, reduce heat to medium-low, cover, and simmer until vegetables are tender, about 20–25 minutes.

4. Stir in the cilantro and season to taste with freshly ground black pepper. Serve immediately.

**Per Serving (1¾ cups)**

| | |
|---|---|
| Calories: 198 | Fiber: 10 grams |
| Fat: 2 grams | Carbohydrates: 35 grams |
| Protein: 11 grams | Sugar: 5 grams |
| Sodium: 39 milligrams | |

# Super Yummy Meatless Meatloaf

**Prep Time:** 10 minutes
**Cook Time:** 20 minutes
**Total Time:** 30 minutes
**Serves 6**

## INGREDIENTS

1 (15-ounce) can no-salt-added kidney beans
1½ cups quick oats
1 small red onion, diced
1 small/medium bell pepper, diced
1 small stalk celery
3 garlic cloves, minced
¼ cup chopped fresh cilantro
1½ teaspoons ground cumin
1 teaspoon salt-free chili seasoning
½ cup low-sodium barbecue sauce, divided
¼ cup salt-free ketchup
3 teaspoons salt-free prepared mustard
Freshly ground black pepper, to taste

Certain to please die-hard meat fans and vegetarians alike, this meatless meatloaf is moist, melt-in-your-mouth comfort food. Pure deliciousness with absolutely no guilt! Make this meatloaf your own and try salt-free salsa instead of ketchup or barbecue sauce, or add in your favorite vegetables and herbs. If you can't find salt-free condiments locally, order them online at *http://healthyheartmarket.com*. Adapted from *The Complete Cooking Light Cookbook*.

1. Preheat oven to 450°F. Spray an 8-inch square pan lightly with oil and set aside.

2. Drain the beans and rinse well. Mash using the tines of a fork and place into a large mixing bowl.

3. Add the oats, onion, bell pepper, celery, garlic, cilantro, cumin, chili seasoning, ¼ cup of the barbecue sauce, ketchup, mustard, and black pepper. Mix together using your hands, then transfer to the prepared pan and smooth to even.

4. Spoon the remaining ¼ cup barbecue sauce over top and spread evenly. Place pan on middle rack in oven and bake for 20 minutes.

5. Remove from oven. Cool briefly before slicing into portions and serving.

**Per Serving (1⅓ cups)**

| | |
|---|---|
| Calories: 227 | Fiber: 9 grams |
| Fat: 2 grams | Carbohydrates: 43 grams |
| Protein: 10 grams | Sugar: 10 grams |
| Sodium: 41 milligrams | |

# Sweet Potatoes Stuffed with Chili

**Prep Time:** 5 minutes
**Cook Time:** 25 minutes
**Total Time:** 30 minutes
**Serves 4**

## INGREDIENTS

4 medium sweet potatoes

2 (15-ounce) cans no-salt-added black beans

¼ cup unsweetened apple juice

1 teaspoon olive oil

1 medium onion, diced

2 cloves garlic, minced

2 medium carrots, sliced

¼ cup low-sodium salsa

1 (14-ounce) can no-salt-added diced tomatoes

½ cup frozen peas

1 tablespoon salt-free chili seasoning

1 teaspoon ground cumin

Freshly ground black pepper, to taste

½ cup nonfat sour cream, optional

### Sweet Potato Facts

Sweet potatoes are often considered holiday fare, something to be enjoyed certain times of the year and forgotten about the rest. But sweet potatoes are a staple we should all be embracing. They're inexpensive and incredibly versatile, adapting to almost any type of cuisine. They're full of vitamins A and C, beta carotene, and super-low in sodium. When buying sweet potatoes, look for firm, orange flesh that's free of soft spots or blemishes. At home, store them in a dark cabinet or drawer, never in the refrigerator.

A flavorful twist on the traditional baked potato, this meatless meal is low in sodium and bursting with tasty veggies. You even can make it vegan by omitting the sour cream. Better yet? This recipe is inexpensive and infinitely variable. Use regular potatoes instead of sweet, add corn instead of peas, substitute kidney beans for black, and so on. Adapted from *Prevention's Low-Fat, Low-Cost Freezer Cookbook*.

1. Scrub the sweet potatoes and pierce all over with the tines of a fork. Place potatoes on a paper towel and/or microwave-safe plate and microwave on high for 7 minutes. Turn potatoes over, then microwave for another 7 minutes.

2. Drain and rinse the black beans and set aside.

3. While the potatoes are cooking, combine the apple juice and olive oil in a sauté pan and bring to a boil over medium heat. Add the onion, garlic, carrots, and salsa and sauté until softened, about 5 minutes.

4. Add the beans, tomatoes (including juice), peas, and seasonings. Reduce heat to low, cover, and cook, stirring frequently, for 20 minutes.

5. Carefully split each cooked sweet potato open and mash slightly. Spoon a quarter of the chili over each sweet potato and top with a dollop of sour cream if desired. Serve immediately.

**Per Serving (1 stuffed sweet potato)**

| | |
|---|---|
| Calories: 493 | Fiber: 18 grams |
| Fat: 2 grams | Carbohydrates: 99 grams |
| Protein: 23 grams | Sugar: 20 grams |
| Sodium: 162 milligrams | |

# Lemon Pesto Rice with Portabella Mushrooms

**Prep Time:** 10 minutes
**Cook Time:** 10 minutes
**Total Time:** 20 minutes
**Serves 6**

## INGREDIENTS

1 tablespoon olive oil

1 large onion, chopped

16 ounces baby bella mushrooms, chopped

6 cups cooked rice (or other grain)

### LEMON PESTO

Juice of 2 fresh lemons

6 cloves garlic

1½ tablespoons olive oil

1½ teaspoons agave nectar

½ teaspoon salt-free prepared mustard

⅓ cup unsalted nuts

⅓ cup fresh basil leaves

2 tablespoons nutritional yeast flakes

1 teaspoon all-purpose salt-free seasoning

Freshly ground black pepper to taste

### For Fun and Freshness, Grow Your Own Herbs!

Fresh herbs are easy and inexpensive to grow in almost any living situation. A sunny windowsill or patio planter can produce enough herbs to flavor a wide array of recipes any time of year. A few bargain pots, some soil, and seeds are all you need to get started. Enjoy your favorite herbs at their freshest by growing your own!

Here's a hearty vegan one-dish meal that's perfect for weeknights and potluck parties. The bright bite of the lemon pesto is amazing in its own right, but with the complementary tastes of sautéed onion, meaty mushrooms, and hearty brown rice, it's downright addictive. This recipe works wonderfully with cooked pasta, as well as quinoa and other grains, so if you're not a huge rice fan, don't let that dissuade you. For the pesto, use your favorite type of unsalted nuts: almonds, walnuts, cashews, or pine nuts.

1. Heat olive oil in a stockpot over medium heat. Add chopped onion and mushrooms and cook, stirring, 10 minutes. Remove from heat, stir in the cooked rice, cover, and set aside.

2. Measure pesto ingredients into a blender or food processor and pulse until smooth.

3. Stir the pesto into the rice mixture until well combined. Season to taste with additional black pepper, if desired. Serve immediately.

**Per Serving (1⅔ cups)**

| | |
|---|---|
| Calories: 324 | Fiber: 4 grams |
| Fat: 10 grams | Carbohydrates: 49 grams |
| Protein: 9 grams | Sugar: 3 grams |
| Sodium: 9 milligrams | |

# Falafel with Tzatziki

**Prep Time:** 10 minutes
**Cook Time:** 20 minutes
**Total Time:** 30 minutes
**Serves 4**

## INGREDIENTS

1 (15-ounce) can no-salt-added garbanzo beans (also called chickpeas)
1 small onion
3 cloves garlic
¼ cup fresh parsley
2 teaspoons ground cumin
1 teaspoon ground coriander
¼ teaspoon dried red pepper flakes
Freshly ground black pepper, to taste

### TZATZIKI

1 small cucumber
2 cloves garlic, finely minced
1 tablespoon chopped fresh dill
1 teaspoon freshly squeezed lemon juice
¾ cup plain nonfat Greek yogurt
All-purpose salt-free seasoning, to taste
Freshly ground black pepper, to taste

These little chickpea patties are such a nice change from the everyday, they'll feel like a special treat. A vegan version of tzatziki can be made using nondairy plain yogurt instead of the regular Greek. Wrap in low-sodium pita or enjoy plain, garnished with extra chopped parsley and fresh chopped tomato.

1. Preheat the oven to 400°F. Spray a baking sheet lightly with oil and set aside.

2. Drain and rinse the chickpeas, then place into a food processor. Add the onion, garlic, parsley, cumin, coriander, dried red pepper flakes, and freshly ground black pepper. Pulse until smooth.

3. Spoon the mixture, tablespoon by tablespoon, onto the prepared baking sheet an inch or two apart. Place sheet on middle rack in oven and bake for 10 minutes. Remove from oven, gently flip falafel patties, and return to bake for another 5–10 minutes.

4. While falafel is baking, peel the cucumber. Slice lengthwise and gently scrape out seeds using a spoon. Grate, then place into a clean towel and squeeze to remove excess liquid.

5. Place into a mixing bowl and add the remaining tzatziki ingredients. Season to taste with salt-free seasoning and freshly ground black pepper and stir well to combine.

6. Remove falafel from oven and serve immediately with tzatziki.

**Per Serving (4 falafel patties and ¼ cup tzatziki)**
Calories: 195
Fat: 3 grams
Protein: 11 grams
Sodium: 15 milligrams
Fiber: 8 grams
Carbohydrates: 22 grams
Sugar: 6 grams

# Quinoa with Mixed Veggies and Cilantro Peanut Pesto

Prep Time: 10 minutes
Cook Time: 15 minutes
Total Time: 25 minutes
Serves 6

## INGREDIENTS

1 cup quinoa

2 cups water

1 teaspoon olive oil

1 medium red onion, diced

2 medium carrots, diced

8 ounces mushrooms, chopped

1 medium red bell pepper, diced

3 tablespoons Cilantro Peanut Pesto (see recipe in this chapter)

2 scallions, sliced

Freshly ground black pepper, to taste

### An Important Note about Quinoa
Quinoa has a bitter-tasting outer coating on its grains that must be removed prior to cooking. Many brands of commercial quinoa remove this prior to packaging, so you can simply measure the quinoa and cook. But if you're not using organic, pre-washed quinoa, don't forget to rinse well prior to cooking.

Creamy, filling, and almost like a quinoa risotto, this hearty one-dish meal has a fabulous combination of flavors. It's a great choice for parties and other group events since it's vegan and uses quinoa, which is a gluten-free grain. For more flavor, simply add additional pesto to the completed dish.

1. Measure the quinoa into a saucepan. Add water and bring to a boil over high heat. Once boiling, reduce heat to medium-low, cover, and simmer for 15 minutes.

2. While the quinoa is cooking, heat the olive oil in a sauté pan over medium heat. Add the onion and sauté for 2 minutes.

3. Add carrots, mushrooms, and bell pepper and cook, stirring, for 8 minutes. Remove from heat.

4. Stir into the cooked quinoa along with the pesto. Sprinkle with the scallions and season to taste with freshly ground black pepper. Serve immediately.

**Per Serving (1½ cups)**
Calories: 204
Fat: 4 grams
Protein: 7 grams
Sodium: 59 milligrams

Fiber: 5 grams
Carbohydrates: 35 grams
Sugar: 5 grams

# Cilantro Peanut Pesto

**Prep Time:** 10 minutes
**Cook Time:** 0 minutes
**Total Time:** 10 minutes
**Yields ½ cup**

## INGREDIENTS

½ cup fresh cilantro
¼ cup light coconut milk
¼ cup unsalted peanuts
4 cloves garlic
Juice and zest of 1 fresh lime

A flavorful change from standard basil pesto or bright lemon pesto, this zesty Asian-inspired sauce tastes great on grains, pasta, and so much more. The pesto calls for peanuts, but other nuts work equally well; I especially love unsalted cashews. Be sure to shake the coconut milk well before opening to get all the yummy goodness off the lid!

1. Place all the ingredients into a food processor and pulse until smooth.

2. Use immediately or store in an airtight container and refrigerate until use.

**Per Serving (2 tablespoons)**

| | |
|---|---|
| Calories: 79 | Fiber: 1 gram |
| Fat: 5 grams | Carbohydrates: 6 grams |
| Protein: 2 grams | Sugar: 2 grams |
| Sodium: 5 milligrams | |

# Red Potatoes with Peas, Parsley, Egg, and Mustard

**Prep Time:** 13 minutes
**Cook Time:** 17 minutes
**Total Time:** 30 minutes
**Serves 4**

## INGREDIENTS

2 large eggs

1½ pounds red potatoes, cut into 1-inch chunks

1 cup fresh or frozen peas

¼ cup dry white wine

1 small onion, chopped

2 tablespoons salt-free prepared mustard

1 tablespoon olive oil

Freshly ground black pepper, to taste

¼ cup chopped fresh parsley

### Parsley Facts

Parsley is an easy-growing herb that comes in two varieties: flat-leaf and curly. It's too often dismissed as a bland plate garnish, but parsley has an amazing, distinctive flavor when eaten raw. Use it to add a refreshing taste and color to salads, dressings, and pastas. Parsley contains high levels of vitamins A, C, and K, as well as antioxidants, and may help prevent cardiovascular disease.

Simple peas and potatoes are elevated to new heights with the addition of mustard, wine, and onion. The chopped hard-boiled egg adds extra protein to this dish, but feel free to eliminate altogether if you're vegan. Served hot or cold, this recipe is excellent in every way. Adapted from the *American Medical Association Family Health Cookbook.*

1. Place the eggs in a small saucepan. Add enough water to cover by an inch. Bring to a boil over high heat. Once boiling, turn off the heat and let the eggs sit for 10–12 minutes before peeling and chopping.

2. While the eggs are cooking, bring a large pot of water to boil, add the potatoes, and cook until tender, roughly 10–15 minutes.

3. If using fresh peas, add them to the boiling water during the last 5 minutes of cooking; if using frozen peas, add 2 minutes before the end.

4. Drain the potatoes and peas into a colander and set aside. Do not wash the pot.

5. Return the pot to the stove, place over high heat, and add the wine and onion. Cook for 1–2 minutes to soften, then remove the pot from the heat and whisk in the mustard, olive oil, and black pepper.

6. Add the potatoes and peas back into the pot along with the chopped eggs, and toss well to coat. Add the parsley and stir. Serve immediately.

**Per Serving (1½ cups)**
Calories: 242
Fat: 5 grams
Protein: 7 grams
Sodium: 40 milligrams

Fiber: 4 grams
Carbohydrates: 38 grams
Sugar: 3 grams

# Speedy Samosa Pasta

**Prep Time:** 10 minutes
**Cook Time:** 15 minutes
**Total Time:** 25 minutes
**Serves 6**

## INGREDIENTS

12 ounces whole-grain angel hair pasta

2 cups frozen peas

2 medium potatoes

1 medium onion

2 cloves garlic, minced

3 tablespoons unsalted butter or olive oil

¼ cup nutritional yeast flakes

1 tablespoon salt-free curry powder

Freshly ground black pepper, to taste

I love Indian samosas and would eat them every day if I had the time to make them. My solution? A pasta version of the classic samosa that whips together in less than 15 minutes. The whole-grain pasta is a nod to the delicious fried dough, but without all the fat. Add in curry powder, sautéed onion, garlic, cooked potato, and peas, and it's all of the flavor, with zero fuss! Use olive oil instead of butter for a delicious vegan version.

1. Cook pasta according to package directions, omitting salt.

2. When there are a few minutes left for the pasta to cook, add the frozen peas to the pot and return to boiling. Once cooked, drain, and return pasta and peas to the pot.

3. While the pasta is cooking, scrub the potatoes and pierce with the tines of a fork. Place potatoes in the microwave and cook roughly 8 minutes, turning once. Once cooked, remove potatoes from microwave, let rest briefly to cool, then dice.

4. While the pasta and potatoes are cooking, heat a small nonstick skillet over medium heat. Add the onion and garlic and cook, stirring, 5 minutes.

5. Add the diced potatoes, onion, and garlic to the pasta and peas. Add the butter (or olive oil) and season with the remaining ingredients. Toss well to coat.

6. Serve immediately.

**Per Serving (1¾ cups)**

| | |
|---|---|
| Calories: 347 | Fiber: 4 grams |
| Fat: 7 grams | Carbohydrates: 60 grams |
| Protein: 13 grams | Sugar: 3 grams |
| Sodium: 46 milligrams | |

# Coconut Cauliflower Curry

**Prep Time:** 5 minutes
**Cook Time:** 25 minutes
**Total Time:** 30 minutes
**Serves 6**

## INGREDIENTS

1 tablespoon canola oil

1 medium onion, diced

6 cloves garlic, minced

1 tablespoon minced fresh ginger

1 tablespoon salt-free garam masala

1 teaspoon ground turmeric

2 tablespoons salt-free tomato paste

2 cups low-sodium vegetable broth

1 cup light coconut milk

1 head cauliflower, cut into florets

3 medium potatoes, diced

2 medium carrots, sliced

1 (15-ounce) can no-salt-added diced tomatoes

1½ cups fresh or frozen peas

½ teaspoon freshly ground black pepper

¼ cup chopped fresh cilantro

The intoxicating array of flavors make this a heavenly vegan meal. Garam masala is a spice blend used extensively in Indian cooking and often contains cinnamon, cumin, coriander, cloves, ginger, nutmeg, pepper, mace, star anise, and bay leaves. It has a potent fragrance and taste, but isn't fiery hot. If you don't have garam masala, you can substitute salt-free curry powder. Serve with steamed brown or basmati rice.

1. Heat oil in a stockpot over medium heat. Add onion, garlic, and ginger and cook, stirring, for 2 minutes.

2. Add the garam masala and turmeric and sauté until fragrant, roughly 30 seconds to 1 minute.

3. Stir in the tomato paste, broth, coconut milk, cauliflower, potatoes, carrots, and tomatoes (including juice) and stir well to combine. Raise heat slightly and bring to a boil. Once boiling, lower heat to medium-low, cover, and simmer for 20 minutes.

4. Stir in the peas and black pepper and cook 2 minutes more.

5. Remove from heat and stir in the cilantro. Serve immediately.

**Per Serving (1½ cups)**
Calories: 178
Fat: 6 grams
Protein: 5 grams
Sodium: 117 milligrams

Fiber: 7 grams
Carbohydrates: 27 grams
Sugar: 11 grams

# Spicy Chickpea Tacos with Arugula

**Prep Time:** 10 minutes
**Cook Time:** 10 minutes
**Total Time:** 20 minutes
**Serves 6**

## INGREDIENTS

1 package low-sodium taco shells

6 cups fresh baby arugula

3 cups cooked no-salt-added garbanzo beans (also called chickpeas)

4 tablespoons salt-free tomato paste

1 (8-ounce) can no-salt-added tomato sauce

1 tablespoon apple cider vinegar

1 tablespoon light brown sugar

2 teaspoons salt-free chili seasoning

1 teaspoon dry ground mustard

1 teaspoon onion powder

½ teaspoon garlic powder

¼–½ teaspoon freshly ground black pepper

⅛–¼ teaspoon dried red pepper flakes

These may just be the tastiest tacos ever! A thick and spicy tomato-based sauce dotted with garbanzos, the peppery cool of arugula, and the crunchy bite of corn—what's not to love? Spoon extra filling over cooked brown rice if you run short of packaged shells. I love arugula for its unique, peppery flavor. If you can't find it, substitute your favorite leafy green instead.

1. Heat taco shells according to package directions.

2. Wash the arugula and pat dry. Set aside.

3. In a saucepan, measure remaining ingredients and stir well to combine.

4. Place pan over medium heat and simmer, stirring frequently, for 10 minutes. Remove from heat.

5. Fill warm taco shells with arugula and spoon bean mixture over top. Serve immediately.

**Per Serving (2 tacos)**
Calories: 288
Fat: 8 grams
Protein: 10 grams
Sodium: 30 milligrams

Fiber: 9 grams
Carbohydrates: 46 grams
Sugar: 10 grams

# CHAPTER 9

# Desserts

Vanilla Cupcakes with Cinnamon-Fudge Frosting

Chocolate Cupcakes with Vanilla Frosting

Chocolate Chip Banana Muffin Top Cookies

Lemon Cookies

Peanut Butter Chocolate Chip Blondies

Ginger Snaps

Carrot Cake Cookies

Chewy Pumpkin Oatmeal Raisin Cookies

Easy Apple Crisp

Mango Crumble

Homemade Banana Ice Cream

Karen's Apple Kugel

Peach Cobbler

Blueberry Pudding Cake

Vegan Rice Pudding

# Vanilla Cupcakes with Cinnamon-Fudge Frosting

**Prep Time:** 10 minutes
**Cook Time:** 18 minutes
**Total Time:** 28 minutes
**Yields 1 dozen**

## INGREDIENTS

1½ cups white whole-wheat flour

¾ cup sugar

¾ teaspoon sodium-free baking powder

½ teaspoon sodium-free baking soda

1 cup nondairy milk

6 tablespoons canola oil

1 tablespoon apple cider vinegar

1 tablespoon pure vanilla extract

### FROSTING

2 cups powdered sugar

⅓ cup unsweetened cocoa powder

4 tablespoons non-hydrogenated vegetable shortening

4 tablespoons nondairy milk

1 teaspoon ground cinnamon

1 teaspoon pure vanilla extract

### Desserts and the DASH Diet

People often equate dieting with deprivation, but sweets can be part of a healthy lifestyle when chosen wisely and consumed in moderation. If you're someone with an above-average sweet tooth, try to channel cravings into the healthy realm of fruit. Keep an array of fresh produce out on the counter and you'll find yourself reaching for it daily. Dried fruit, applesauce, and juice-sweetened fruit cups also make great guilt-free treats.

Fast, delicious, and foolproof, these vegan cupcakes are perfect for any occasion. Feel free to swap out the vanilla extract for your favorite flavors. Lemon, almond, and maple are all delicious alone or partnered with the pure vanilla. I adore this thick cinnamon-infused chocolate frosting, but the cupcakes work equally well with other flavors. Get creative with different combinations and find the ones you like best!

1. Preheat oven to 350°F. Line a 12-muffin tin with paper liners and set aside.

2. Measure the flour, sugar, baking powder, and baking soda into a mixing bowl and whisk well to combine. Add the remaining batter ingredients and stir just until combined.

3. Divide the batter evenly between the muffin cups. Place tin on middle rack in oven and bake 18 minutes.

4. Remove cupcakes from oven and place on wire rack to cool.

5. Measure the frosting ingredients into a clean mixing bowl and beat until fluffy.

6. Frost cupcakes. Serve immediately or cover until ready to serve.

**Per Serving (1 cupcake)**

| | |
|---|---|
| Calories: 347 | Fiber: 4 grams |
| Fat: 7 grams | Carbohydrates: 60 grams |
| Protein: 13 grams | Sugar: 3 grams |
| Sodium: 46 milligrams | |

# Chocolate Cupcakes with Vanilla Frosting

**Prep Time:** 10 minutes
**Cook Time:** 20 minutes
**Total Time:** 30 minutes
**Yields 1 dozen**

## INGREDIENTS

1½ cups white whole-wheat flour

1 cup sugar

2 teaspoons sodium-free baking soda

¼ cup unsweetened cocoa powder

1 cup water

4 tablespoons canola oil

4 tablespoons unsweetened applesauce

1 tablespoon pure vanilla extract

1 teaspoon distilled white vinegar

### FROSTING

1½ cups powdered sugar

4 tablespoons non-hydrogenated vegetable shortening

2½ tablespoons nondairy milk

1 tablespoon pure vanilla extract

Cholesterol-free cupcakes for chocolate lovers. For low-fat cupcakes, substitute applesauce for all of the oil in the batter and top with powdered sugar instead of frosting. For a slightly different twist on the recipe, feel free to add any of the following to the batter: a ½ cup of chocolate chips, unsweetened shredded coconut, chopped nuts, or dried or fresh fruit.

1. Preheat oven to 350°F. Line a 12-muffin tin with paper liners and set aside.

2. Measure the flour, sugar, and baking soda into a mixing bowl and whisk well to combine. Add the remaining batter ingredients and stir just until combined.

3. Divide the batter evenly between the muffin cups. Place tin on middle rack in oven and bake 20 minutes or until toothpick inserted in center of cupcakes comes out clean.

4. Remove cupcakes from oven and place on wire rack to cool.

5. Measure the frosting ingredients into a clean mixing bowl and beat until fluffy.

6. Frost cupcakes. Serve immediately or cover until ready to serve.

**Per Serving (1 cupcake)**

Calories: 272

Fat: 9 grams

Protein: 2 grams

Sodium: 2 milligrams

Fiber: 1 gram

Carbohydrates: 45 grams

Sugar: 32 grams

# Chocolate Chip Banana Muffin Top Cookies

**Prep Time:** 5 minutes
**Cook Time:** 15 minutes
**Total Time:** 20 minutes
**Yields 16 cookies**

## INGREDIENTS

1 cup quick oats

1 cup white whole-wheat flour

¼ cup sugar

1 tablespoon sodium-free baking powder

1 teaspoon ground cinnamon

3 ripe medium bananas, mashed

4 tablespoons canola oil

1 tablespoon pure vanilla extract

¾ cup chocolate chips

### Cut the Fat!

When looking to minimize oil in baked goods, try substituting unsweetened applesauce, mashed banana, or puréed prunes for all or part of the fat. When sautéing, coat the bottom of pans with water or fat-free low-sodium broth. Little steps like this add up, and will keep you slimmer and healthier.

These delicious muffin top cookies make fabulous guilt-free snacks any time of the day! Soft, sweet, and totally addictive, these cookies are mostly fruit-sweetened and low in refined sugar. I love the added boost of the chocolate chips, but you may omit them if you'd prefer. Adapted from *Vive le Vegan!*

1. Preheat oven to 350°F. Line a baking sheet with parchment paper and set aside.

2. Measure the oats, flour, sugar, baking powder, and cinnamon into a mixing bowl and whisk well to combine. Add the remaining ingredients and stir just until combined.

3. Using a medium-sized ice cream scoop, scoop the batter onto the prepared baking sheet, leaving an inch or two between cookies. Place the baking sheet on middle rack in oven and bake 15 minutes.

4. Remove from oven and place on wire rack to cool.

5. Serve immediately or store in an airtight container.

**Per Serving (1 cookie)**

Calories: 150

Fat: 6 grams

Protein: 2 grams

Sodium: 0 milligrams

Fiber: 1 gram

Carbohydrates: 23 grams

Sugar: 10 grams

# Lemon Cookies

**Prep Time:** 5 minutes
**Cook Time:** 10 minutes
**Total Time:** 15 minutes
**Yields 3 dozen**

## INGREDIENTS

2½ cups white whole-wheat flour
1½ cups sugar
1 tablespoon sodium-free baking powder
¾ cup canola oil
Juice and grated zest of 2 large lemons
1 tablespoon pure vanilla extract

Crisp, buttery, and cholesterol-free, these deliciously simple cookies shine with bright citrus flavor. If you don't have fresh lemons on hand, substitute ½ cup bottled lemon juice. You can also swap out the fresh lemons for limes, oranges, or grapefruits for added fun and interest. Adapted from Food.com.

1. Preheat oven to 350°F.

2. Measure the flour, sugar, and baking powder into a mixing bowl and whisk well to combine. Add the remaining ingredients and stir to form a stiff dough.

3. Drop by rounded tablespoons onto an ungreased baking sheet. Place sheet on middle rack in oven and bake 10 minutes.

4. Remove from oven and let cool on sheet for a few minutes before transferring to a wire rack to cool fully.

5. Serve immediately or store in an airtight container.

**Per Serving (1 cookie)**

| | |
|---|---|
| Calories: 106 | Fiber: 0 grams |
| Fat: 5 grams | Carbohydrates: 15 grams |
| Protein: 1 gram | Sugar: 8 grams |
| Sodium: 0 milligrams | |

# Peanut Butter Chocolate Chip Blondies

**Prep Time:** 5 minutes
**Cook Time:** 20 minutes
**Total Time:** 25 minutes
**Yields 2 dozen**

## INGREDIENTS

¼ cup salt-free peanut butter

¾ cup light brown sugar

½ cup unsweetened applesauce

¼ cup canola oil

2 egg whites

1 tablespoon pure vanilla extract

2 teaspoons sodium-free baking powder

1 cup unbleached all-purpose flour

½ cup white whole-wheat flour

½ cup semisweet chocolate chips

### Cookie Baking Tip

When baking cookie bars, allow them to cool fully in the pan before slicing and removing. This keeps the edges intact and helps ensure your cookie bars look picture perfect. To get evenly sized bars, slice halfway through the pan, then divide each half in half, and slice again.

Peanut butter and chocolate form a mouthwatering combination in this dense, moist cookie bar. For an equally delicious vegan version, whisk together 2 tablespoons of egg replacement powder or 2 tablespoons of ground flaxseed with 6 tablespoons of water in a small bowl. Let the mixture rest for a few minutes and then add it to the batter instead of the egg whites. For extra flavor and crunch, sprinkle some chopped unsalted peanuts on top of the batter before baking.

1. Preheat oven to 400°F. Grease and flour a 9" × 13" baking pan and set aside.

2. Measure the peanut butter, sugar, applesauce, oil, egg whites, and vanilla into a mixing bowl and stir well to combine.

3. Add the baking powder and mix.

4. Gradually add in the flours, stirring well.

5. Fold in the chocolate chips.

6. Spread batter in prepared pan and smooth to even. Place pan on middle rack in oven and bake for 20 minutes. Remove from oven and place on wire rack to cool.

7. Cool before cutting into bars and serving.

**Per Serving (1 cookie bar)**

| | |
|---|---|
| Calories: 18 | Fiber: 1 gram |
| Fat: 5 grams | Carbohydrates: 17 grams |
| Protein: 2 grams | Sugar: 10 grams |
| Sodium: 7 milligrams | |

# Ginger Snaps

## INGREDIENTS

4 tablespoons unsalted butter

½ cup light brown sugar

2 tablespoons molasses

1 egg white

2½ teaspoons ground ginger

¼ teaspoon ground allspice

1 teaspoon sodium-free baking soda

½ cup unbleached all-purpose flour

½ cup white whole-wheat flour

1 tablespoon sugar

Fans of classic ginger snaps will love biting into these dark, aromatic cookies! They're not only low in sodium, but they're also low in fat, too! For an even richer flavor, add a tablespoon or two of brewed coffee to the batter—rich espresso works particularly well. I also like adding a little bit of ground cardamom for balance.

1. Preheat oven to 375°F. Line a baking sheet with parchment paper and set aside.

2. Place the butter, sugar, and molasses into a mixing bowl and beat well to combine.

3. Add the egg white, ginger, and allspice and mix well.

4. Stir in the baking soda, then gradually add the flours. Beat until combined, scraping down the sides of the bowl as necessary.

5. Scoop the dough by tablespoons and roll into small balls. Place balls on lined baking sheet and press down using a glass dipped in the tablespoon sugar. Once the glass presses on the dough, it will moisten sufficiently to coat with sugar.

6. Place baking sheet on middle rack in oven and bake for 10 minutes.

7. Remove from oven and transfer cookies to a wire rack to cool. Store in an airtight container.

**Per Serving (1 cookie)**

| | |
|---|---|
| Calories: 81 | Fiber: 0 grams |
| Fat: 2 grams | Carbohydrates: 14 grams |
| Protein: 1 gram | Sugar: 8 grams |
| Sodium: 6 milligrams | |

# Carrot Cake Cookies

**Prep Time:** 10 minutes
**Cook Time:** 12 minutes
**Total Time:** 22 minutes
**Yields 3 dozen**

## INGREDIENTS

3 medium carrots, shredded

1½ cups white whole-wheat flour

¾ cup oat flour

¾ cup light brown sugar

1 egg white

⅓ cup canola oil

1 tablespoon pure vanilla extract

1 teaspoon sodium-free baking powder

1½ teaspoons ground cinnamon

½ teaspoon ground nutmeg

¼ teaspoon ground ginger

⅛ teaspoon ground cloves

### Ice Cream Scoops Make Perfect Cookies!

Instead of fumbling with tablespoons, scoop out cookie dough using a small retractable ice cream scoop. Ice cream scoops produce uniform, picture-perfect cookies and reduce hassle and mess. Small scoops are sold at kitchenware shops and other stores as well as online.

Soft whole-grain cookies with the taste and texture of carrot cake. For more carrot cake flavor, feel free to add some chopped unsalted walnuts, raisins, or unsweetened shredded coconut. Don't have packaged oat flour? No problem! Make it at home by measuring rolled oats into a food processor and pulsing until fine.

1. Preheat oven to 375°F. Line a baking sheet with parchment paper and set aside.

2. Place all the ingredients into a mixing bowl and stir well to combine. Dough will be quite sticky.

3. Drop by tablespoons onto lined baking sheet. Place sheet on middle rack in oven and bake for 12 minutes.

4. Remove from oven and transfer cookies to a wire rack to cool. Store in an airtight container.

**Per Serving (1 cookie)**

Calories: 67

Fat: 2 grams

Protein: 1 gram

Sodium: 7 milligrams

Fiber: 0 grams

Carbohydrates: 10 grams

Sugar: 4 grams

# Chewy Pumpkin Oatmeal Raisin Cookies

Prep Time: 4 minutes
Cook Time: 16 minutes
Total Time: 20 minutes
Yields 4 dozen

## INGREDIENTS

1 cup pumpkin purée

1⅔ cups sugar

2 tablespoons molasses

1½ teaspoons pure vanilla extract

⅔ cup canola oil

1 tablespoon ground flaxseed

2 teaspoons Ener-G Baking Soda Substitute

1 teaspoon ground cinnamon

½ teaspoon ground nutmeg

1 cup unbleached all-purpose flour

1 cup white whole-wheat flour

1⅓ cups rolled or quick oats

1 cup seedless raisins

Irresistibly chewy and fabulously flavorful, these oatmeal raisin cookies are made even better by the addition of pumpkin! Soft, sweet, and amazingly delicious, you'll find yourself eating them by the handful, so watch out. High in heart-healthy omega-3s, ground flaxseed is sold in many supermarkets and health food stores alongside the baking supplies or in the bulk bins. It's fairly perishable because of the oil in the seeds, so be sure to seal it well and store in the freezer; ground flaxseed meal will keep well for weeks when frozen. Adapted from *Vegan with a Vengeance*.

1. Preheat oven to 350°F. Spray 2 baking sheets lightly with oil and set aside.

2. Measure the ingredients into a large mixing bowl and stir together using a rubber spatula, scraping the bottom and sides of the bowl to incorporate everything fully.

3. Scoop batter out by tablespoons—a small retractable ice cream scoop works wonderfully here—and place on the prepared baking sheets.

4. Place sheets on middle rack in oven and bake 16 minutes. Remove from oven and transfer cookies to a wire rack to cool.

5. Repeat process with remaining batter. Once cool, store cookies in an airtight container.

**Per Serving (1 cookie)**
Calories: 97
Fat: 3 grams
Protein: 1 gram
Sodium: 1 milligram
Fiber: 0.6 grams
Carbohydrates: 16 grams
Sugar: 9 grams

# Easy Apple Crisp

**Prep Time:** 5 minutes
**Cook Time:** 25 minutes
**Total Time:** 30 minutes
**Serves 8**

## INGREDIENTS

6 medium apples

1 tablespoon lemon juice

⅓ cup sugar

½ cup rolled or quick oats

½ cup white whole-wheat flour

½ cup light brown sugar

1 tablespoon pure vanilla extract

1 teaspoon ground cinnamon

½ teaspoon ground ginger

3 tablespoons unsalted butter

Juicy fruit under a sweet whole-grain crust. What's not to love? This fabulous crisp is a perfect vehicle for fall fruit. Vary the apples for different tastes and textures. Tart varieties, such as Granny Smiths, retain their shape much better than their softer, sweeter siblings. For interest, substitute pears for the apples, add raisins, dried or fresh cranberries to the filling, or chopped nuts to the crust. For a cholesterol-free vegan version, use coconut oil or non-hydrogenated shortening instead of the butter.

1. Preheat oven to 425°F. Take out a 2-quart baking pan and set aside.

2. Peel and core the apples and slice each into 16 wedges.

3. Place into a mixing bowl, add the lemon juice and sugar, and toss well to coat.

4. Turn mixture out into the baking pan and set aside.

5. Place the oats, flour, sugar, vanilla, and spices into a mixing bowl and stir to combine.

6. Cut the butter into the mixture using your hands and process until a wet crumb has formed. Sprinkle mixture over the fruit.

7. Place pan on middle rack in oven and bake for 25 minutes. Remove from oven and place on a wire rack to cool.

**Per Serving (1 cup)**
Calories: 232
Fat: 5 grams
Protein: 2 grams
Sodium: 5 milligrams

Fiber: 2 grams
Carbohydrates: 46 grams
Sugar: 34 grams

# Mango Crumble

**Prep Time:** 5 minutes
**Cook Time:** 25 minutes
**Total Time:** 30 minutes
**Serves 8**

## INGREDIENTS

2 barely ripe mangoes

2 tablespoons light brown sugar

1 tablespoon cornstarch

1½ teaspoons minced fresh ginger

½ cup unbleached all-purpose flour

½ cup white whole-wheat flour

½ cup sugar

1 teaspoon ground cinnamon

¼ teaspoon ground ginger

3 tablespoons unsalted butter

Sink your teeth into tender chunks of mango and a cinnamon-scented crust. For a juicier filling, omit the cornstarch. Can't find mangoes? Substitute 2 cups fresh or canned pineapple chunks, peaches, blueberries, strawberries, or another favorite fruit instead. This is delicious served warm or cool, dolloped with nonfat or low-fat frozen yogurt.

1. Preheat oven to 375°F. Take out an 8-inch square baking pan and set aside.

2. Peel mangoes and cut into 1-inch chunks. Place in a mixing bowl.

3. Add the brown sugar, cornstarch, and minced ginger and toss to coat. Turn mixture out into the baking pan and spread to even.

4. In another bowl, whisk together the flours, sugar, cinnamon, and ginger.

5. Cut the butter into small pieces and add to the bowl. Work butter into the mixture using your hands until it resembles damp sand and sticks together when squeezed. Sprinkle mixture evenly over the fruit.

6. Place pan on middle rack in oven and bake for 25 minutes, until fruit is tender. Remove from oven and place on wire rack to cool. Serve warm or cool.

**Per Serving (½ cup)**

Calories: 190
Fat: 5 grams
Protein: 3 grams
Sodium: 3 milligrams

Fiber: 2 grams
Carbohydrates: 37 grams
Sugar: 23 grams

# Homemade Banana Ice Cream

**Prep Time:** 2 minutes
**Cook Time:** 0 minutes
**Total Time:** 2 minutes
**Serves 4**

## INGREDIENTS

4 ripe bananas

**Homemade Vegan Chocolate Shell**
If you love the taste and texture of that magical chocolate shell sold in stores and ice cream parlors, here's how to make your own at home! Simply measure ½ cup chocolate chips into a microwave-safe bowl or mug, add 1 teaspoon canola oil, and microwave for 1 minute. Stir until smooth and drizzle over your favorite frozen dessert. It hardens almost instantly, like magic!

This dessert contains only one ingredient: bananas! Yet when frozen and puréed, the crystallized fruit so perfectly mimics the look, taste, and texture of soft-serve ice cream, that it's almost magic. Peel the bananas before freezing to make this the easiest dessert ever created. And for an even tastier treat, make your very own vegan chocolate shell—recipe in sidebar!

1. Place bananas in freezer and freeze until solid.

2. Remove bananas from freezer, peel, and slice into chunks. Place chunks into a blender or food processor and pulse until smooth.

3. Scoop mixture out and serve immediately.

**Per Serving (½ cup)**
Calories: 105
Fat: 0 grams
Protein: 1 gram
Sodium: 1 milligram

Fiber: 3 grams
Carbohydrates: 26 grams
Sugar: 14 grams

# Karen's Apple Kugel

**Prep Time:** 5 minutes
**Cook Time:** 25 minutes
**Total Time:** 30 minutes
**Serves** 8

## INGREDIENTS

3 sheets unsalted matzo

2 cups water

4 tart green apples

1 tablespoon freshly squeezed lemon juice

3 tablespoons unsalted butter, melted

¼ cup brown sugar

½ cup seedless raisins

3 egg whites

1½ teaspoons ground cinnamon

### What Is Matzo?

Matzo is a type of unleavened bread, traditionally composed of only flour and water. Although associated with the Jewish Passover holiday, matzo can be purchased year round in most places, and is typically stocked in the kosher section of the supermarket. Matzo have a large cracker-like appearance and often contain little or no sodium, making them a terrific base for peanut butter and jelly sandwiches, Swiss cheese, hummus, and more.

A healthy dessert that also makes a great holiday side dish or simple breakfast. The softened matzo gives this kugel a creamy texture and appearance without additional fat, cholesterol, or sodium. The recipe was given to me years ago by a lovely friend from Philadelphia. Many thanks to Karen for sharing!

1. Preheat oven to 400°F. Take out an 8" × 11" baking dish and set aside.

2. Place the matzo in an 8-inch square baking pan. Pour the water into the pan and set aside to rehydrate.

3. Peel apples, core, and cut into quarters. Cut each quarter crosswise into thirds, and then lengthwise into slices no more than ¼ inch thick. Transfer apples to a mixing bowl.

4. Check on the matzo. When soft, drain the matzo and squeeze out excess water.

5. Place matzo into the mixing bowl. Add the remaining ingredients and stir well to combine.

6. Pour mixture into the 8" × 11" baking dish. Place dish on middle rack in oven and bake for 25 minutes.

7. Remove from oven. Set on a wire rack to cool. Cut into portions and serve warm or cool.

**Per Serving (1 cup)**

| | |
|---|---|
| Calories: 181 | Fiber: 2 grams |
| Fat: 4 grams | Carbohydrates: 34 grams |
| Protein: 3 grams | Sugar: 21 grams |
| Sodium: 24 milligrams | |

# Peach Cobbler

**Prep Time:** 5 minutes
**Cook Time:** 25 minutes
**Total Time:** 30 minutes
**Serves 8**

## INGREDIENTS

6 ripe peaches, peeled and sliced

3 tablespoons sugar

Juice of 1 fresh lemon

1¼ cups unbleached all-purpose flour

½ cup white whole-wheat flour

⅔ cup sugar

1 teaspoon sodium-free baking powder

4 tablespoons unsalted butter, melted and cooled

1 egg white

½ cup low-fat milk

1 tablespoon pure vanilla extract

An updated version of the classic dessert with heart-healthy whole grain and ripe, juicy fruit. When fresh peaches are out of season, substitute two 15-ounce cans instead. Look for peaches packed only in fruit juice—not syrup—and drain well. Serve with whipped cream and/or nonfat frozen yogurt if desired.

1. Preheat oven to 425°F. Take out a 9" × 13" baking dish and set aside.

2. Place sliced peaches into a mixing bowl, add sugar and lemon juice and toss well to coat. Transfer to the baking dish. Set aside.

3. Measure the flours, sugar, and baking powder into a mixing bowl and whisk well to combine.

4. Add the melted butter, egg white, milk, and vanilla and stir well to combine. Batter will be thick. Spoon batter over sliced peaches.

5. Place baking dish on middle rack in oven and bake for 25 minutes.

6. Remove dish from oven and place on wire rack to cool. Serve warm or cool.

**Per Serving (1 cup)**
Calories: 273
Fat: 6 grams
Protein: 5 grams
Sodium: 15 milligrams

Fiber: 3 grams
Carbohydrates: 50 grams
Sugar: 28 grams

# Blueberry Pudding Cake

Prep Time: 5 minutes
Cook Time: 25 minutes
Total Time: 30 minutes
Serves 6

## INGREDIENTS

3 cups blueberries

¾ cup sugar, divided

1 tablespoon freshly squeezed lemon juice

6 tablespoons unsalted butter, softened

2 teaspoons pure vanilla extract

1 teaspoon freshly grated lemon zest

1 egg white

1½ teaspoons sodium-free baking powder

2 tablespoons low-fat milk

⅔ cup white whole-wheat flour

### Blueberry Facts

Blueberries have been harvested for thousands of years in North America, and are an easy garden crop, requiring only acidic soil and adequate rainfall. Blueberries are high in vitamins K and C as well as manganese, and contain several antioxidants believed to inhibit cancer and inflammation. Fresh blueberries make a delicious addition to baked goods, salads, and sauces, but they are also fairly perishable. To prevent spoilage, freeze blueberries and thaw as needed.

Living in Maine, I am blessed by many things. Abundant snow in winter, majestic coastline in summer, and in fall, a bumper crop of wild blueberries you wouldn't believe. This homey dessert is simply heaven in a bowl. Luscious berries oozing into a soft, semisolid cake. When fresh blueberries are out of season, frozen ones work just as well. Enjoy warm or cold, topped with low-fat whipped cream if desired.

1. Preheat oven to 400°F. Spray an 8-inch square baking pan lightly with oil and set aside.

2. Place blueberries into a mixing bowl. Add ¼ cup sugar and the lemon juice and toss well to coat.

3. Pour berries into the prepared baking pan, place on middle rack in oven, and bake for 5 minutes. Remove from oven and set aside.

4. Place the butter and remaining ½ cup sugar into a mixing bowl and beat to combine.

5. Add the vanilla, lemon zest, and egg white and mix well.

6. Add the baking powder and milk and stir. Gradually add in the flour, mixing until combined.

7. Pour batter over the cooked blueberries. Place pan on middle rack in oven and bake for 20 minutes, until golden brown.

8. Remove from oven and place pan on wire rack to cool. Serve warm or cool.

**Per Serving (¾ cup)**

| | |
|---|---|
| Calories: 300 | Fiber: 2 grams |
| Fat: 12 grams | Carbohydrates: 46 grams |
| Protein: 2 grams | Sugar: 32 grams |
| Sodium: 14 milligrams | |

# Vegan Rice Pudding

**Prep Time:** 5 minutes
**Cook Time:** 20 minutes
**Total Time:** 25 minutes
**Serves 8**

## INGREDIENTS

1 quart vanilla nondairy milk
1 cup basmati or jasmine rice, rinsed
¼ cup sugar
1 teaspoon pure vanilla extract
⅛ teaspoon pure almond extract
½ teaspoon ground cinnamon
⅛ teaspoon ground cardamom

You don't need dairy to make some of the most delicious pudding in the world—I mean it! You may not believe me, but this recipe produces a delicious vegan rice pudding that's thick and creamy, with just a hint of the exotic. The pudding thickens significantly as it cools; if you prefer a thinner consistency, stir in a little nondairy milk before serving.

1. Measure all of the ingredients into a saucepan and stir well to combine. Bring to a boil over medium-high heat.

2. Once boiling, reduce heat to low and simmer, stirring very frequently, about 15–20 minutes.

3. Remove from heat and cool. Serve sprinkled with additional ground cinnamon if desired.

**Per Serving (¼ cup)**
Calories: 148
Fat: 2 grams
Protein: 4 grams
Sodium: 48 milligrams
Fiber: 1 gram
Carbohydrates: 26 grams
Sugar: 10 grams

# CONVERSION CHARTS

## VOLUME CONVERSIONS

| U.S. Volume Measure | Metric Equivalent |
|---|---|
| ⅛ teaspoon | 0.5 milliliter |
| ¼ teaspoon | 1 milliliter |
| ½ teaspoon | 2 milliliters |
| 1 teaspoon | 5 milliliters |
| ½ tablespoon | 7 milliliters |
| 1 tablespoon (3 teaspoons) | 15 milliliters |
| 2 tablespoons (1 fluid ounce) | 30 milliliters |
| ¼ cup (4 tablespoons) | 60 milliliters |
| ⅓ cup | 90 milliliters |
| ½ cup (4 fluid ounces) | 125 milliliters |
| ⅔ cup | 160 milliliters |
| ¾ cup (6 fluid ounces) | 180 milliliters |
| 1 cup (16 tablespoons) | 250 milliliters |
| 1 pint (2 cups) | 500 milliliters |
| 1 quart (4 cups) | 1 liter (about) |

## WEIGHT CONVERSIONS

| U.S. Weight Measure | Metric Equivalent |
|---|---|
| ½ ounce | 15 grams |
| 1 ounce | 30 grams |
| 2 ounces | 60 grams |
| 3 ounces | 85 grams |
| ¼ pound (4 ounces) | 115 grams |
| ½ pound (8 ounces) | 225 grams |
| ¾ pound (12 ounces) | 340 grams |
| 1 pound (16 ounces) | 454 grams |

## OVEN TEMPERATURE CONVERSIONS

| Degrees Fahrenheit | Degrees Celsius |
| --- | --- |
| 200 degrees F | 95 degrees C |
| 250 degrees F | 120 degrees C |
| 275 degrees F | 135 degrees C |
| 300 degrees F | 150 degrees C |
| 325 degrees F | 160 degrees C |
| 350 degrees F | 180 degrees C |
| 375 degrees F | 190 degrees C |
| 400 degrees F | 205 degrees C |
| 425 degrees F | 220 degrees C |
| 450 degrees F | 230 degrees C |

## BAKING PAN SIZES

| American | Metric |
| --- | --- |
| 8 × 1½ inch round baking pan | 20 × 4 cm cake tin |
| 9 × 1½ inch round baking pan | 23 × 3.5 cm cake tin |
| 11 × 7 × 1½ inch baking pan | 28 × 18 x 4 cm baking tin |
| 13 × 9 × 2 inch baking pan | 30 × 20 × 5 cm baking tin |
| 2 quart rectangular baking dish | 30 × 20 × 3 cm baking tin |
| 15 × 10 × 2 inch baking pan | 30 × 25 × 2 cm baking tin (Swiss roll tin) |
| 9 inch pie plate | 22 × 4 or 23 × 4 cm pie plate |
| 7 or 8 inch springform pan | 18 or 20 cm springform or loose bottom cake tin |
| 9 × 5 × 3 inch loaf pan | 23 × 13 × 7 cm or 2 lb narrow loaf or pate tin |
| 1½ quart casserole | 1.5 liter casserole |
| 2 quart casserole | 2 liter casserole |

# INDEX